*This book is dedicated to my children, Michael Matthew Orrison,
Jennifer Jean Orrison, and William Werner Orrison, III, and to my
wife, Rebecca Lynn Spiller Orrison.
Without your help, there would be no book!*

Contents

Preface

This atlas is intended to serve as a reference and guide to the various structures of the human brain, and to the function that each of these structures performs.

The text is divided into five sections. The first section provides a basis for understanding the function or functional relationships of the various brain structures via a glossary of the neuroanatomic terminology that includes a detailed description of each structure. If the exact function of a given structure is uncertain, a description of the known connections or closely associated structures is provided. These definitions are referenced so that the reader may consult the original source for more information or additional references. In each of the remaining sections of the atlas, which comprise drawings as well as CT and MR scans, summary definitions are provided along with references. For immediate access to an expanded definition the reader can consult the glossary in the first section of the text. A section on 3D imaging is included because this is becoming a more frequently utilized form of image display.

As the emphasis on studying and imaging of the human brain shifts from anatomy and pathology to function, it becomes increasingly important for us to know what functional role the various parts of the brain may play. Even the most rudimentary attempts at functionally imaging the brain, or correlating neuroanatomy with function, require a basic understanding of where to look in the brain for a given function. As our methods of evaluation improve, so will the details that can be contained in texts such as this.

Functional brain imaging is a relatively new area of clinical medicine, as well as a significant advance in basic neuroscience research. In this decade of the brain, it serves as one of the most exciting and valuable breakthroughs in our understanding of the human mind. As the applications of functional brain imaging expand, we are beginning to appreciate the importance of understanding not only how the brain looks, but also what it is actually doing. Brain function is beginning to be analyzed in ways never before deemed possible, and it is the cognitive functions that intrigue us the most. Can we really know what dreams are made of, from whence comes imagination, creativity, or even despair? For those involved in functional imaging of the brain, there are, for now, far more questions than answers. Some of the answers are contained in this text. However, our understanding of the human mind is increasing at an unprecedented rate. Consequently, this guide to understanding the structural and functional relationships of the human mind is just that, a guide. As the reader's level of knowledge increases, so will the need for consulting additional and perhaps updated references.

I acknowledge the many individuals who have contributed to the completion of this text, especially my wife, Rebecca L. Orrison, R.N., whose dedication to the completion of this project actually made it possible. Her endless hours of typing as well as checking and cross-checking references and definitions have enhanced the final product immensely. Thanks also go to Mary Espinosa, R.N., who provided the administrative support that resulted in a finished product. I am also indebted to Stephany Scott, Senior Editor, whose patience, support, and friendship throughout this project made the entire process most favorable. Mike Norviel, Mary Grebenc, and Lisa Ordonez provided drawings and anatomic identifiers that formed the basis for much of the material presented. I am very appreciative of the many hours of hard work by Carol Garner, who produced the final drawings that are used throughout the book, and special thanks to Jim Janis, who provided the photography. I also wish to thank Jonathan Briggs, our department editor; Sheila Mulligan-Webb, division editor; and staff for their help. Dr. John Sanders and Jonathan Stearley provided formatted images. Dr. Blaine Hart reviewed the structural and functional relationships. Dr. Jeffrey Lewine reviewed the functional definitions and provided updated information as required. Drs. Fred A. Mettler, Jr. and Michael F. Hartshorne have provided an academic atmosphere within our department that makes the pursuit of projects such as this both possible and enjoyable.

A dedicated clinical and support staff enabled the acquisition of the images and editing of the written text. They are Mike Caress, Mike Davis, Brian Dorotik, Todd Ellis, Geneva Ham, Kim McGonigle, Herman Mettling, Jeff Meyer, Joe Monasterio, Pedro Quiroga, Joanna Stein, Sheila Rhodus, Dan Williamson, and Vardaman Wash.

William W. Orrison, Jr., M.D.

Glossary of Structures
and Definitions

Abducens nerve (cranial nerve VI). The abducens nerve, cranial nerve VI, is a motor nerve that innervates the lateral rectus muscle of the eye. The lateral rectus provides for outward (lateral) movements of the eye.[1 (p. 104)]

Abducens nucleus (VI). Located in the lower pons, the abducens nucleus contains the cell bodies of the motor neurons that give rise to the abducens nerve. These motor neurons control outward movements of the eye, through their innervation of the lateral rectus muscle. The abducens nucleus, along with the oculomotor, trochlear, and hypoglossal nuclei, forms the general somatic motor column of the brainstem.[1 (p. 404), 2 (p. 322–330)]

Accessory nerve (cranial nerve XI, spinal accessory nerve). Cranial nerve XI, the spinal accessory nerve, is a motor nerve composed of spinal and cranial roots. The spinal root contains motor fibers that innervate the sternocleidomastoid and trapezius muscles that provide for movement of the head and shoulders. Fibers of the cranial root originate in the nucleus ambiguus of the medulla. Together with fibers of the vagus nerve, fibers of the cranial root innervate muscles of the pharynx and larynx.[2 (p. 322–330)]

Accessory nucleus (XI). The accessory nucleus gives rise to the spinal root of cranial nerve XI, the spinal accessory nerve. Nerve XI mediates movements of the head and shoulders. The cells of the accessory nucleus are found at the medullary level, extending inferiorly from the level of the pyramidal decussation down to the 5th cervical segment.[2 (p. 322–330)]

Accessory olivary nuclei. The accessory olivary nuclei, in conjunction with the principal olivary nucleus, forms a structure known as the inferior olivary complex (nucleus). The olivary complex receives its input from the spinal cord, the ipsilateral red nucleus, the contralateral cerebellum, and both cerebral hemispheres. The olive gives rise to climbing fiber input to the contralateral cerebellum, through the inferior cerebellar peduncle. The inferior olivary complex plays an important role in sensory motor integration and coordination.[3 (p. 203)]

Alveolar process of the maxilla. One of the four processes of the maxilla (alveolar, frontal, palatine, and zygomatic), the alveolar process contains eight sockets for the teeth and is the origin of the buccinator muscle.[4 (p. 338–340)]

Ambient cistern. The ambient cistern is a CSF-containing subarachnoid space surrounding the mesencephalon.[5 (p. 116)]

Amygdala (amygdaloid complex). The amygdaloid complex is part of the limbic system, and is a heterogeneous collection of small nuclear groups located in the anterior dorsomedial aspect of the temporal lobe. It is divided into two main nuclear groups: the corticomedial group and the basolateral group. The amygdala demonstrates reciprocal connections with the thalamus, basal ganglia, hypothalamus, temporal cortex, and septal and preoptic areas. It is involved in modulation of multiple functions, including olfaction, emotive behavior, and integration of visceral activity.[2] (pp. 200–202)

Angle of the mandible.   The angle is formed by the junction of the body and ramus of the mandible. It is the region of insertion of the masseter and medial pterygoid muscles.[4] (p. 316)

Angular gyrus.   Located in the inferior parietal lobule, the angular gyrus is believed to be involved in visual-auditory integration. Lesions of the angular gyrus of the dominant hemisphere (usually the left) result in a disruption of receptive language abilities.[6] (pp. 18–20), [7] (pp. 405–407)

Ansa lenticularis.   This fiber pathway is formed by neuronal connections from the internal segment of the globus pallidus to the ventral anterior and ventral lateral thalamic nuclei, and is involved in motor function.[2] (pp. 281–282)

Anterior arch of the atlas (C1).   The anterior arch is formed by the joining of the lateral masses of the first cervical vertebrae.[4] (pp. 273–274), [8] (pp. 129–130)

Anterior belly of the digastric muscle.   The digastric muscle is one of the muscles of the floor of the mouth. It is comprised of anterior and posterior bellies joined by an intermediate tendon that is connected to the body and greater horn of the hyoid bone by a loop of fibrous connective tissue. This loop forms a pulley that raises and steadies the hyoid bone during swallowing and speech. The anterior belly arises from the inner surface of the mandible, just beneath the mylohyoid muscle.[9] (pp. 665–667)

Anterior cerebral artery.   The anterior cerebral artery is the branch of the external carotid artery that supplies orbital and medial aspects of the frontal lobe. It also supplies medial aspects of the parietal lobe.[7] (p. 59), [10] (p. 191)

Anterior commissure.   The anterior commissure is a bundle of 2 to 3 million fibers that interconnect right and left temporal cortices. It provides for the interhemispheric exchange of information. Some efferent connections between one anterior olfactory nucleus and the contralateral olfactory bulb cross the midline as part of the anterior commissure.[11] (p. 246), [12] (pp. 249–250)

Anterior horn of the lateral ventricle.   The anterior horn of the lateral ventricle lies in the frontal lobe, anterior to the interventricular foramen. Like other portions of the ventricular system, it is an ependymal-lined cavity filled with CSF. The anterior horn is typically void of CSF-producing choroid plexus.[1] (172–173), [11] (p 283), [12] (p. 253–256)

Anterior lobe of the pituitary.   The anterior lobe of the pituitary, the adenohypophysis, produces a wide range of hormones, including growth hormone, thyroid-stimulating hormone, follicle-stimulating hormone, luteinizing hormone, corticotropin (ACTH), and prolactin. Release of these hormones is under control of hypothalamic nuclei that send neurosecretory fibers onto the vasculature of the median eminence. Releasing and inhibiting factors are secreted into the hypophyseal portal system, which carries these factors to the anterior lobe.[2] (p. 350), [3] (pp. 421–424), [12] (pp. 201–203)

Anterior perforated substance.   The anterior perforated substance is a region near the optic chiasm where branches of the anterior cerebral artery perforate into the brain to supply the basal ganglia and internal capsule. The olfactory tubercle, a collection of neurons that send efferent projections to the olfactory bulb, is found in the anterolateral aspects of the anterior perforated substance.[2] (pp. 200–202)

Arachnoid granulations.   Arachnoid granulations are clusters of arachnoid villi within the superior sagittal sinus. Arachnoid villi are the main site of reabsorption of CSF into the venous system.[2] (p. 100)

Arcuate fasciculus.   The arcuate fasciculus is a fiber bundle interconnecting Wernicke's receptive and Broca's expressive language areas. Lesions of this pathway cause a conduction aphasia.[2] (p. 184)

Atlas (C1).   The atlas, the first cervical vertebrae, is comprised of two lateral masses joined anteriorly and posteriorly by arches. Unlike other vertebrae, the atlas lacks a body, with that position occupied by the odontoid process (dens) of the second vertebral body (axis), around which the atlas rotates.[4] (pp. 273–274), [8] (pp.129–130)

Auditory cortex.   Located on the dorsal surface of the superior temporal gyrus, the primary auditory cortex shows tonotopic organization for the processing of sound information. It receives input from the medial geniculate nucleus of the thalamus and projects to surrounding auditory association areas.[2] (pp. 182–184)

Auditory nerve (vestibulocochlear nerve, cranial nerve VIII).   The auditory nerve is a branch of the vestibulocochlear nerve, cranial nerve VIII. The vestibulocochlear nerve is divided into vestibular and cochlear subdivisions, both of which transmit information from specialized inner ear receptors to brainstem nuclei. The cochlear division of the auditory nerve carries information from hair cells of the organ of Corti (located in the cochlea) to the cochlear nuclei (located at the level of the pontomedullary junction). The vestibular division carries vestibular information from hair cells in the semicircular canals to vestibular nuclei of the rostral medulla and caudal pons.[13] (pp. 245–246)

Auditory nucleus (VIII) (cochlear).   This nucleus consists of two divisions, the dorsal and ventral cochlear nuclei, with both divisions projecting to the inferior colliculus. These nuclei are important in localizing and recognizing patterns of sound.[2] (pp. 166–167)

Auditory nucleus (VIII) (vestibular).   This is part of the vestibular nuclear complex, which consists of four nuclei in the rostral medulla and caudal pons. The major projections are to brainstem nuclei involved in the control of extraocular muscles and to the spinal cord through the vestibulospinal tracts. This nucleus is involved in transmitting information regarding equilibrium.[2] (p. 167), [3] (p. 199)

Auricle.   The auricle is the extracranial portion of the external ear. It consists of a thin plate of elastic cartilage covered by skin. The auricle collects and funnels vibratory information to the middle ear.[14] (p. 167)

Axis (C2).   The axis, the second cervical vertebrae, is distinguished by the odontoid process (dens) that serves as a pivot for C1, the atlas. The body has an anterior elongation that overlaps the superior body of C3 and serves as the attachment for the anterior longitudinal ligament. This large and powerful spinous process absorbs the pull of the head and neck muscles that extend, retract, and rotate the head.[4] (pp. 273–274), [8] (pp. 129–130)

Basal ganglia.   The basal ganglia is a collection of subcortical nuclei involved in regulation of motor function and with an additional possible role in cognitive functioning. The basal ganglia include the caudate nucleus, the lenticular nucleus (which is comprised of the putamen and globus pallidus), the subthalamic nucleus, and the substantia nigra.[6] (p. 304), [7] (p. 11)

Basilar artery.   The basilar artery is formed by the merging of the left and right vertebral arteries (which ascend along the spinal column and lower medulla) at the upper medullary level. The basilar artery supplies blood to the upper medulla, pons, cerebellum, inner ear, occipital lobe, and part of the temporal lobe. At the level of the pontine-midbrain junction, it bifurcates into left and right posterior cerebral arteries.[15] (p. 1042)

Basis pedunculi (crus cerebri).   Located at the level of the mesencephalon (midbrain), the basis pedunculi are formed by the descending projections of the pyramidal and corticopontine systems that descend from the cortex through the internal capsule, basis pedunculi, and medullary pyramids. The descending fibers demonstrate a somatotopic arrangement with the face, arm, trunk, and leg represented sequentially from medial to lateral aspects of the basis pedunculi.[2] (pp. 224–225), [12] (p. 116)

Body of the corpus callosum.   The corpus callosum is divided into the rostrum, genu, body, and splenium, and is the largest of the forebrain commissures. The body contains interhemispheric fibers connecting left and right parietal, temporal, and posterior frontal regions, including the sensorimotor cortices. It provides for interhemispheric transfer of sensory and cognitive information.[2] (pp. 51, 131), [12] (p. 248), [16] (33)

Body of the mandible. The body of the mandible is the horizontal portion of the mandible that is shaped like a bent horseshoe. From this, an ascending process (the ramus) runs upward. Together, the body and ramus form the lower jaw and face. The mandible contains 16 cavities for the lower teeth.[8] (pp. 121–123), [17] (p. 815)

Body of the tongue. The posterior root, the tip, and the body make up the tongue. The main function of the tongue is to squeeze food into the pharynx for swallowing and to aid in the formation of words during speech. The tongue is the site of taste buds, which are collections of specialized epithelial cells sensitive to certain chemicals.[9] (p. 745)

Broca's area. Located on the frontal operculum at the opercular and triangular ports of the inferior frontal gyrus, Broca's area (Brodmann's area 46) is critically involved in language production. This region displays significant functional asymmetry with the left opercular region generally playing a more critical language role than the right. Lesions of Broca's area of the dominant hemisphere produce an expressive aphasia.[2] (p. 184)

Calcar avis. The calcar avis is a white matter eminence in the posterior horn of the lateral ventricle that is caused by the calcarine sulcus on the medial surface of the occipital lobe.[10] (pp. 74–75)

Calcarine sulcus. The calcarine sulcus demarcates upper and lower visual field representations in the striate, primary visual cortex of the occipital lobe. The upper visual field is represented in the lower calcarine cortex, and vice versa.[2] (pp. 217–218), [11] (pp. 242, 260)

Callosal sulcus. The callosal sulcus lies just above the corpus callosum and below the cingulate gyrus.[11] (p. 236)

Carotid canal. The carotid canal opens into the foramen lacerum and provides for entry of the internal carotid artery into the skull.[9] (p. 680)

Caudate nucleus. The caudate nucleus is an elongated subcortical mass that is part of the basal ganglia. It is a C-shaped structure with its head contiguous with the anterior perforated substance, its body curving and lying adjacent to the inferior border of the anterior horn of the lateral ventricle. The body tapers posteriorly and inferiorly to form the tail, which enters the roof of the temporal horn of the lateral ventricle to end at the level of the amygdala. The caudate receives input from rostral areas of the cerebral cortex, sensorimotor cortex, the intralaminar nuclei of the thalamus, and the substantia nigra. It projects back to the substantia nigra and also to the globus pallidus, which in turn projects to the anterior and lateral ventral nuclei of the thalamus. These thalamic nuclei project to frontal and prefrontal cortical areas. The caudate is involved in motor function and possibly in certain cognitive functions.[6] (p. 304), [7] (p. 11), [12] (pp. 207–212), [15] (pp. 306–307), [18] (pp. 523–524)

Central sulcus. The central sulcus runs downward and forward across the lateral cerebral surface and divides the parietal and frontal lobes. The anterior bank is formed by Brodmann's area 4, the primary motor cortex of the precentral gyrus. The posterior bank is formed by Brodmann's area 3b, part of the primary somatosensory cortex of the postcentral gyrus.[19] (p. 257)

Central tegmental tract. This tract passes through the reticular formation carrying both afferent and efferent fibers. Of particular note are descending projections from the red nucleus to the ipsilateral inferior olivary nucleus. Ascending fibers from the gustatory nucleus to the ipsilateral ventral posterior medial nucleus of the thalamus are also contained in this tract.[2] (p. 193), [6] (p. 162)

Centromedian nucleus. One of six intralaminar nuclei of the thalamus, the centromedian nucleus receives input from other thalamic nuclei and projects to the striatum and insular taste cortex.[12] (p. 184), [20] (p. 263)

Centrum semiovale. This refers to the superior

radiations of the internal capsule. It is composed of commissural, projection, and cortical association fibers.[13] (p. 86)

Cerebellar hemisphere. The lateral aspect of the cerebellum is involved with movements of the proximal and distal extremities. It provides neuronal projections through the dentate nucleus and the contralateral ventrolateral thalamic nucleus to the contralateral precentral gyrus for the control of fine, coordinated movements. The net motor influence of each cerebellar hemisphere is on ipsilateral musculature because of the decussation of descending motor fibers from the precentral gyrus.[7] (p. 283), 12 (p. 175), 15 (pp. 633–634)

Cerebellar tonsil. Located just off of the midline, the cerebellar tonsils along with the cerebellar vermis make up the spinocerebellum. This region of the cerebellar cortex receives its input from the spinocerebellar tracts. It influences limb movement and posture through descending projections to the globose and fastigial nuclei.[2] (p. 242)

Cerebellar vermis. This is the midline portion of cerebellum that regulates and coordinates axial and girdle musculature. The vermis receives spinocerebellar input as well as vestibular, visual, and auditory input relayed by brainstem nuclei. Its primary efferent projections are to the globose and fastigial nuclei. It also influences attention, sensation, motivation, memory, behavior, and autonomic activities.[3] (p. 282), 7 (p. 290)

Cerebellum. Located within the posterior cranial fossa, and consisting of a cortex (gray matter) arranged in transverse folds (folia), a medullary center (white matter), and four pairs of central nuclei (1, fastigial; 2, globose; 3, emboliform; and 4, dentate), this complex structure is primarily involved in motor function through the maintenance of equilibrium and the coordination of muscle action.[1] (pp. 15, 132–133), 4 (pp. 338–340), 7 (pp. 18–20)

Cerebral aqueduct (aqueduct of Sylvius). A central cavity that traverses the midbrain connecting the third and fourth ventricles, this provides a pathway for CSF to leave the third ventricle and enter the fourth ventricle. Obstruction at this level of the ventricular system is a common cause of hydrocephalus.[2] (p. 22), 11 (p. 213)

Cerebral peduncle. These structures are formed by the sides of the midbrain excluding the tectum. They include the tegmentum (which contains the red nucleus and substantia nigra) and also the basis pedunculi (which contain the corticospinal tracts that at this level are arranged medial to lateral as face, arm, trunk, and leg).[2] (p. 226), 12 (p. 108)

Chiasmatic cistern. This is one of the ventral CSF-filled subarachnoid spaces about the brain. It merges posteriorly above the sella turcica with the interpeduncular cistern and anteriorly with the cistern of the lamina terminalis. It is bounded medially above by the optic chiasm and the pituitary stalk, and laterally above by the anterior perforated substance. This cistern is continuous laterally with the cistern of the sylvian fissure.[10] (pp. 113–120)

Choroid plexus. The choroid plexus is a vascular fringelike fold of pia mater involved in the production of CSF.[5] (p. 102), 14 (p. 1213)

Of fourth ventricle. Within the fourth ventricle, it is attached on the ventricular side of the posterior medullary velum under the nodule and lingula of the vermis of the cerebellum.[5] (p. 102), 14 (p. 1213)

Of third ventricle. Within the third ventricle, it is attached to the undersurface of the velum interpositum, which extends from the foramen of Monro posteriorly the full length of the ventricle.[5] (p. 102), 14 (p. 1213)

Of lateral ventricle. The choroid plexus extends throughout the lateral ventricle, and at all levels of the ventricular system it is involved in the production of CSF.[5] (p. 102), 14 (p. 1213)

Choroid fissure. This is a CSF-containing space between the fimbria of the hippocampus and diencephalon to which the choroid plexus is attached. It forms a portion of the medial wall of the lateral ventricle.[1] (pp. 19, 172–173), 12 (pp. 255, 267)

Cingulate gyrus. This is a part of the limbic system that plays a role in emotional behavior, the regulation of the autonomic nervous system, learning, and memory. It receives input from medial, dorsal, and anterior thalamic nuclei, and it projects back to the cortex and the parahippocampal gyrus through the cingulum.[12] (p. 272), [18] (pp. 255, 674)

Cingulate sulcus. This sulcus separates the cingulate gyrus from the superior frontal gyrus on the medial surface of the hemispheres.[19] (p. 261)

Claustrum. A thin sheet of gray matter that separates the external capsule from the subcortical white matter, it may be involved in mediating visual attention.[11] (p. 244), [15] (p. 460)

Clivus of sphenoid bone. A bony surface extending from the foramen magnum to the dorsum sellae with the lower part formed as part of the basilar occipital bone and the upper part from the body of the sphenoid bone, it supports the medulla oblongata and the lower pons.[4] (p. 320), [14] (p. 328)

Cochlea (acoustic labyrinth). This is the auditory part of the inner ear, and one of the three parts of the osseous labyrinth (the other two being the vestibule and the semicircular canals). The cochlea is composed of a central bony portion (modiolus), which contains the cochlear (spiral) ganglion within the snail-like spiral shell of two and a half turns. Within the labyrinth is the organ of Corti (the transduction site of sound energy into neural signals). This is the primary organ of hearing.[1] (p. 254); [8] (pp. 374–375, 379), [14] (p. 334)

Collateral eminence. The collateral eminence is a shallow prominence of white matter in the floor of the trigone of the lateral ventricle (secondary to the collateral fissure on the undersurface of the temporal lobe).[10] (pp. 74–75)

Collateral sulcus. Located on the ventral surface of the brain, this sulcus, along with its anterior extension, the rhinal sulcus, forms the lateral margin of the limbic association cortex.[2] (pp. 378–379)

Column of the fornix. This structure is part of a myelinated pathway that connects the hippocampus with subcortical structures.[11] (p. 276), [12] (pp. 268–269), [19] (p. 269)

Cornea. This avascular transparent circular anterior outer fibrous layer of the eyeball is largely responsible for refraction of the light that enters the eye.[9] (p. 714)

Corona radiata. This radiating fan of projection fibers from the internal capsule to every part of the cerebral cortex consists of reciprocal connections between the cerebral cortex and the thalamus.[12] (p. 251), [14] (p. 361)

Corpus callosum. The callosum is the largest brain commissure (fiber path). Divided from anterior to posterior into four parts (rostrum, genu, body, and splenium), the callosum interconnects the cerebral hemispheres. It supports the interhemispheric exchange of learned discriminations, and sensory and mnemonic information.[2] (p. 131), [12] (p. 248), [16] (p. 33), [21] (p. 4)

Cribriform plate. This is the horizontal plate of the ethmoid bone, which with the perpendicular plate and the two lateral masses (labyrinths) forms the roof of the nasal fossa as well as part of the floor of the cranial cavity.[4] (pp. 334–336), [8] (p. 119)

Crista galli. This is the midline projection from the cribriform plate into the cranial cavity and serves as an attachment for the falx cerebri.[22] (p. 124)

Crural cistern. The crural cistern is a subarachnoid space filled with CSF. It is a lateral extension of the interpeduncular cistern around the cerebral peduncles through which the posterior communicating artery passes.[10] (p. 117)

Crus of fornix. This structure is part of a myelinated pathway that connects the hippocampus with subcortical structures.[11] (p. 276), [12] (pp. 268–269), [19] (p. 269)

Cuneate fasciculus. This is an ascending fiber pathway carrying somatosensory (touch and proprioceptive) information from the upper extremities to the dorsal column nuclei. Along with the gracile fasciculus, it forms the dorsal columns, which have an orderly somatotopic organization with the leg, trunk, arm, and neck represented from medial to lateral.[2] (pp. 121–122), [3] (p. 203)

Cuneate nucleus. Located at the level of the lower medulla, the cuneate nucleus is the first major relay in the ascending pathway for touch discrimination and proprioception from the upper extremities. It contains synaptic interactions for lateral inhibition that allows for more discrete localization. The gracile and cuneate nuclei together are referred to as the dorsal column nuclei. Relay cells of the cuneate nucleus project to the contralateral thalamus via the medial lemniscus.[2] (pp. 121–122), [3] (p. 203)

Cuneus. The cuneus is also referred to as the "cuneate gyrus" and is separated from the inferior lingual gyrus by the calcarine sulcus. The cortical aspects of the cuneate and the lingual gyri constitute the primary visual cortex and together are called the calcarine or striate cortex.[1] (pp. 160–161)

Dentate gyrus. One of the three components of the hippocampal formation (along with the subiculum and the hippocampus proper), the dentate gyrus occupies the space between the fimbria of the hippocampus and the parahippocampal gyrus. The dominant input to the dentate gyrus is from entorhinal cortex via the perforant pathway. The dentate is characterized by a densely packed layer of small granular cells that give rise to the mossy fiber system that projects to hippocampal pyramidal cells. The hippocampal formation is involved in memory and the emotions related to survival, including visceral and motor responses of reproduction and defense.[2] (p. 379), [12] (pp. 266–267), [13] (pp. 325–326)

Dentate nucleus. The largest of the four deep cerebellar nuclei (dentate, emboliform, globose, and fastigial), the dentate receives projections from the cerebellar cortex and pontocerebellar fibers. It projects to the contralateral ventrolateral nucleus of the thalamus, which then projects primarily on to the premotor cortex and the primary motor cortex. Some dentate projections terminate on the contralateral red nucleus. Through these routes, the dentate modulates somatic motor activity.[1] (pp. 353–354)

Digastric muscle. A straplike muscle with two bellies joined by an intermediate tendon connected to the body and greater horn of the hyoid bone by a loop of fibrous connective tissue. The connective tissue forms a pulley, raising the hyoid bone and steadying it during swallowing and speech. These muscles also depress the mandible.[8] (pp. 121–123), [17] (p. 815)

Diploic space. A space between the two tables of the cranial bones that is filled with loose osseous tissue.[14] (p. 450)

Dorsal trigeminothalamic tract. Similar to the spinothalamic tract, this tract courses through the midbrain to the thalamus transmitting ipsilateral touch and pressure sensations from the face.[2] (p. 307), [3] (p. 193)

Dorsomedial nucleus. The most medial nucleus of the thalamus, which with the anterior nucleus forms the limbic functional division of the thalamic nuclei, this nucleus receives input from the basal lateral amygdala, prefrontal cortex, and the periventricular hypothalamus. It projects to the orbital frontal and prefrontal cortices and is involved with memory and emotion.[12] (p. 184), [20] (p. 263)

Dorsum sellae. This structure forms the posterior boundary of the sella turcica, and projects above with a posterior clinoid process on each side. Decalcification of the dorsum sellae is one of the early signs of an increase in intracranial pressure on plain skull x-rays.[9] (pp. 645–650)

Emboliform nucleus. One of the four cerebellar nuclei (emboliform, dentate, globose, and fastigial), the emboliform nucleus receives input from paramedian areas of the cerebellar cortex. It projects to the contralateral red nucleus and contralateral ventral lateral thalamic nucleus. Together with the globose nucleus, the emboliform nucleus forms the interposed nuclear complex. The interposed nuclei preferentially modulate motor functions of the red nucleus.[2] (p. 242), [6] (pp. 350–353), [20] (pp. 322–329)

Ethmoid air cells. These air cells are contained within the ethmoid bone between the nose and orbit. They drain into the infundibulum, are lined with mucoperiosteum, and are filled with air. They communicate with the nasal cavity and act as resonators to the voice.[23] (pp. 734–736)

Ethmoid bone. This bone forms the roof of the

nasal fossa as well as part of the floor of the cranial cavity and consists of four parts: horizontal (cribriform) plate, peduncular plate, and two lateral masses (labyrinths).[4 (pp. 334–336), 8 (p. 119)]

Eustachian tube (auditory tube, pharyngotympanic tube). This is a connection between the tympanic cavity and the nasopharynx that equalizes air pressure in the middle ear with atmospheric pressure, allowing free movement of the tympanic membrane.[9 (p. 772), 14 (p. 1625)]

External auditory (acoustic) meatus. This is the outer opening of the ear, consisting of a cartilaginous lateral third and an osseous medial two thirds. It forms an S-shaped curve and contains ceruminous glands for the secretion of ear wax (cerumen). The cerumen prevents skin maceration and discourages insects. The warm, humid air within this meatus is essential for the effective mechanical responses of the tympanic membrane.[4 (p. 1192)]

External capsule. This thin sheet of white matter forms the lateral boundary of the lentiform nucleus and consists mainly of association fibers, projection fibers, and commissural fibers.[2 (p. 276), 12 (p. 209), 13 (p. 79)]

External occipital protuberance. This is a median projection of the occipital bone with the central-most prominent projection called the inion. It forms the superior limit of the posterior aspect of the neck.[9 (p. 637)]

Extreme capsule. A thin layer of white matter containing corticocortical association fibers, the extreme capsule separates the claustrum from the insula.[2 (p. 276), 12 (p. 209)]

Facial nerve (cranial nerve VII). Consisting of motor and sensory (intermediate) parts, this nerve supplies the face. The motor root provides innervation to the muscles of the face, scalp, auricle, the buccinator, platysma, stapedius, stylohyoid, and posterior belly of the digastric. The intermediate root transmits taste from the anterior two thirds of the tongue and the soft palate. It also provides preganglionic parasympathetic (secretomotor) innervation to the submandibular and sublingual glands, the lacrimal gland, and the nasal and palatine mucosal glands.[1 (pp. 416–419), 4 (p. 1070)]

Facial nucleus. One of four cranial nerve nuclei within a brainstem nuclear column. The column is comprised of the trigeminal motor nucleus, the facial motor nucleus, the nucleus ambiguus, and the accessory nucleus. This nucleus contains motor neurons that innervate the muscles of facial expression. Cortical projections to the facial nucleus are such that muscles of the upper face are under bilateral control from the motor cortex, whereas muscles of the lower face are under control of the contralateral motor cortex.[2 (pp. 322–333)]

Falx cerebri. The falx cerebri is formed by the fold of right and left dural coverings into the deep midline interhemispheric (longitudinal) cerebral fissure that separates the cerebral hemispheres.[19 (pp. 21, 491)]

Fastigial nucleus. Associated with the vestibular system and receiving projections from the vestibulocerebellum, the vestibular labyrinth, and the vestibular nuclei, this deep cerebellar nucleus sends projections to the lateral and inferior vestibular nuclei and to the pontine and medullary reticular formation. It modulates the vestibulospinal system and the corticoreticulospinal system affecting postural and proximal limb movement.[1 (pp. 352–354)]

Foramen magnum. The largest foramen of the skull, it is located at the most inferior margin of the posterior cranial fossa and connects the cranial cavity with the spinal canal. The medulla, vertebral arteries, spinal roots of the accessory (XI) nerves, dural veins, anterior and posterior spinal arteries, and the meninges pass through this foramen.[9 (pp. 680–681)]

Foramen of Magendie. This is a single midline aperture located in the posterior medullary velum in the inferior roof of the fourth ventricle. Along with the paired lateral foramina of Luschka, it serves as an outlet of the ventricular system to the subarachnoid space.[1 (p. 174), 14 (p. 117)]

Foramen of Monro. These are paired, short canals interconnecting the lateral ventricles of the brain with the midline unpaired third ventricle.[1 (p. 172)]

Foramen ovale. This is an opening through the greater wing of the sphenoid bone through which the third division of the trigeminal nerve (V^3, the mandibular nerve) and the accessory meningeal artery pass.[9 (p. 680)]

Foramina of Luschka (foramina of Key and Retzius). These are paired openings at the ends of the lateral recesses of the fourth ventricle that, with the single midline foramen of Magendie, are the only outlets of the ventricular system to the subarachnoid space.[1 (p. 174), 14 (p. 117)]

Forceps major (forceps occipitalis). This structure consists of the splenium of the corpus callosum and the associated white matter radiations that interconnect the occipital lobes.[12 (p. 248)]

Forceps minor (forceps frontalis). This structure consists of the genu of the corpus callosum and the white matter radiations that interconnect the frontal lobes.[12 (p. 248)]

Fornix. The fornix is the largest efferent tract of the hippocampus. It contains more than a million nerve fibers projecting to the mamillary bodies of the hypothalamus. Beginning as the alveus (thin white matter covering the hippocampus), efferent fibers from the hippocampus converge to form the fimbria of the fornix. The fiber bundle ascends to form the crus of the fornix, which curves around the posterior thalamus, where it is joined by the crus from the opposite side to form the body of the fornix. The body is closely applied to the inferior corpus callosum and is joined anteriorly to the corpus callosum by the septum pellucidum. At the junction of the crus of the fornix are transverse fibers called the commissure of the fornix, which connect the two sides of the hippocampi. The body separates anteriorly into the columns, which curve anteriorly and inferiorly over the foramen of Monro, with each column laterally transversing the wall of the third ventricle to reach the mamillary bodies. Lesions of the fornix disrupt mnemonic functions.[11 (p. 276), 12 (p. 268–269), 19 (p. 269)]

Fourth ventricle. The fourth ventricle is a CSF-filled cavity that is located at the level of the brainstem. It is connected to the third ventricle via the cerebral aqueduct. CSF leaves the fourth ventricle by way of two lateral apertures (foramen of Luschka) and one median aperture (foramen of Magendie). It is continuous inferiorly with the central canal of the medulla oblongata and the spinal cord.[7 (p. 70), 13 (p. 97)]

Frenulum of tongue. A mucous membrane arranged vertically under the tongue, attaching it to the floor of the mouth.[14 (p. 619)]

Frontal bone. This bone forms the anterior cranial vault. It includes the forehead and extends posteriorly over the top of the skull to the coronal suture meeting the right and left parietal bones. It provides enclosure and protection of the brain.[24 (p. 170)]

Frontal lobe. Located superior to the sylvian fissure and anterior to the central sulcus, the frontal lobe contains four prominent functional areas (prefrontal cortex, Broca's area, premotor area, and primary motor cortex). The prefrontal cortex is involved in mnemonic functions and other higher cognitive functions related to personality, insight, and foresight. Located in the inferior frontal gyrus, Broca's area (on the dominant side) is involved in the production of spoken language. Premotor areas (including the supplementary motor area) are involved in the initiation and sequencing of voluntary movements. Located along the anterior bank of the central sulcus, the primary motor cortex of the precentral gyrus gives rise to descending pyramidal fibers that control voluntary movements. This cortical region displays somatotopy in the form of an inverted homunculus (foot at the top and face at the bottom).[6 (pp. 18–20)]

Frontal process of zygomatic bone. This bone forms the lateral margin of the orbit. It articulates with the frontal bone at the lateral border of the superior orbit.[20 (p. 655)]

Frontal sinuses. These are paired air cavities located in the frontal bone on either side and separated by a bony septum. They communicate with the middle meatus of the nasal cavity on the same side. Along with the other sinuses, they act as a resonator to the voice.[9 (pp. 760–762), 14 (p. 1424), 23 (pp. 734–736)]

Fusiform gyrus (lateral occipitotemporal gyrus).   Located on the inferior surface of the brain, this gyrus consists of a visual association cortex. It is divided from the medial occipitotemporal gyrus by the occipitotemporal sulcus and is continuous with the inferior temporal gyrus. This region of the brain contains high-order visual association areas that mediate spatial vision and visual mnemonic and attentional processes.[2] (pp. 156–157), [12] (223, 235–236), [14] (p. 674)

Genioglossus muscle.   This muscle is one of the three extrinsic muscles of the tongue. It originates on the superior medial spine of the mandible and inserts on the undersurface of the tongue and the body of the hyoid bone. It serves to retract, depress, and protrude the tongue as well as to elevate the hyoid bone.[4] (p. 1304), [8] (pp. 204–205, 257)

Genu of corpus callosum.   The genu is the anterior enlargement of the corpus callosum that contains commissural fibers interconnecting the frontal lobes. It tapers inferiorly into the rostrum. The genu and associated white matter radiations to the frontal lobes form the forceps frontalis (forceps minor).[2] (pp. 51, 131), [12] (p. 248), [15] (p. 365), [19] (p. 269)

Globe.   Located in the anterior orbit, the globe contains the cornea, sclera, anterior chamber, and iris of the eye.[8] (pp. 380–384), [25] (p. 188)

Globose nucleus.   One of the four cerebellar nuclei (emboliform, dentate, globose, and fastigial), the globose nucleus receives input from the vermis of the cerebellum. It projects to the contralateral red nucleus and contralateral ventral lateral thalamic nucleus. Together with the emboliform nucleus, the globose nucleus forms the interposed nuclear complex. The interposed nuclei preferentially modulate motor functions of the red nucleus.[2] (p. 242), [6] (pp. 350–353), [20] (pp. 322–329)

Globus pallidus.   Together with the putamen, the globus pallidus forms the lenticular nucleus of the basal ganglia. The lenticular nucleus in conjunction with the caudate forms the corpus striatum, the functional part of the basal ganglia involved in the control of movement.

The globus pallidus receives input from the caudate nucleus, the putamen, the substantia nigra, and the subthalamic nucleus of the basal ganglia. It projects to the anterior and lateral nuclei of the thalamus, the subthalamic nucleus, and midbrain tegmental areas. Through these pathways, it modulates somatic motor functions.[6] (p. 306), [7] (p. 11), [20] (pp. 276–277)

Glossopharyngeal nerve (cranial nerve IX).   This is a mixed nerve that contains afferent fibers that convey taste, touch, pain, and temperature sensations from the tongue, and efferent fibers that innervate muscles of the pharynx. This nerve emerges from the brainstem as a series of five or six nerve rootlets just dorsal to the inferior olive.[1] (p. 420), [20] (pp. 244–246)

Gracile fasciculus.   This is an ascending fiber pathway carrying somatosensory (touch and proprioceptive) information from the lower extremities to the dorsal column nuclei. Along with the cuneate fasciculus, it forms the dorsal columns, which have an orderly somatotopic organization with the leg, trunk, arm, and neck represented from medial to lateral.[2] (pp. 121–122), [3] (p. 203)

Gracile nucleus.   Located at the level of the lower medulla, the gracile nucleus is the first major relay in the ascending pathway for touch discrimination and proprioception from the lower extremities. It contains synaptic interactions for lateral inhibition that allows for more discrete localization. The gracile and cuneate nuclei together are referred to as the dorsal column nuclei. Relay cells of the gracile nucleus project to the contralateral thalamus via the medial lemniscus.[2] (pp. 121–122), [3] (p. 203)

Great cerebral vein (vein of Galen).   This unpaired midline venous structure is formed by the two internal cerebral veins as they enter the quadrigeminal cistern. The great cerebral vein crosses the quadrigeminal cistern in the midline and follows underneath the splenium of the corpus callosum, extending superiorly where it joins the straight sinus at the junction of the falx and the tentorium. It is part of the deep encephalic venous system assisting in venous drainage of the brain.[10] (pp. 275–294)

Habenular commissure. This commissure is located in the dorsal wall of the pineal stalk and contains fibers of the stria medullaris thalami with interconnections between the habenular nuclei. The habenular commissure and the habenular nuclei commonly demonstrate calcification on computed tomography (CT) or plain skull x-rays.[2 (pp. 194–195), 3 (p. 165)]

Habenular nuclei. Along with the pineal gland, the habenular nuclei and their connections form the epithalamus. The habenular nuclei give off bundles of fibers known as the habenulointerpeduncular fasciculus (fasciculus retroflexus of Meynert) that project to the interpeduncular nucleus of the midbrain and through the reticular formation to influence the hypothalamus. Left and right habenular nuclei are interconnected by the habenular commissure. The habenular commissure and the habenular nuclei commonly demonstrate calcification on CT or plain skull x-rays. [2 (pp. 194–195), 3 (p. 165)]

Hard palate. Formed by the palatine processes of the maxillae and the horizontal plates of the palatine bones, the hard palate and the soft palate form the roof of the mouth. The hard palate supports the floor of the nasal cavity.[4 (p. 1270), 8 (p. 467)]

Hippocampus. One of the major components of the limbic system, the hippocampus plays an important role in learning and memory, emotional behavior, and regulation of the autonomic nervous system. Its main source of input is from the entorhinal cortex (via the perforant pathway); dominant output is to the mamillary bodies via the fornix. Bilateral lesions of the hippocampus and associated parahippocampal regions cause significant memory deficits. The hippocampus is particularly prone to epileptic activity.[15 (p. 307), 16 (pp. 630–631), 18 (pp. 255–256), 20 (pp 342–347)]

Hypoglossal nerve (cranial nerve XII). The hypoglossal is the motor nerve of the tongue. It has only a general somatic efferent component. It provides innervation to the musculature of the tongue.[1 (p. 429), 4 (p. 1083)]

Hypoglossal nucleus. The hypoglossal nucleus is located in the midline of the medulla immediately below the floor of the fourth ventricle. The axons exit the nucleus between the inferior olive and the medullary pyramids as a row of small fascicles, which collate to form the hypoglossal nerve. It is the fourth member of the general somatic motor column (oculomotor nucleus, trochlear nucleus, abducens nucleus, and hypoglossal nucleus) and contains the motor neurons projecting peripherally through the hypoglossal nerve to innervate the intrinsic muscles of the tongue.[2 (pp. 322–333)]

Hypothalamus. The hypothalamus together with the thalamus forms the diencephalon lying between the cerebral hemispheres and the midbrain. The hypothalamus is positioned immediately below the thalamus and it forms the floor and lower lateral walls of the third ventricle. The hypothalamus is a collection of nuclear groups that regulate the autonomic nervous system and visceral as well as motivational functions. Example functions are temperature regulation, water balance, feeding and drinking behavior, and sexual activity. It also controls pituitary function via neuronal links to the posterior lobe and a vascular connection to the anterior lobe. There are extensive afferent and efferent connections to the thalamus, midbrain, and limited cerebral cortex.[3 (pp. 421–424)]

Indusium griseum. This structure covers the dorsal surface of the body of the corpus callosum and contains a thin layer of gray matter with two strands of fibers on each side. These are called the medial and lateral longitudinal striae and proceed from the medial olfactory area to the hippocampus.[12 (p. 248)]

Inferior cerebellar peduncle. This structure connects the cerebellum to the medulla. It contains primarily afferent axons entering the cerebellum from the caudal pons, and efferent fibers from the fastigial nucleus to the vestibular nuclei. These pathways are important in maintaining equilibrium. The peduncles form the lateral walls of the fourth ventricle.[2 (p. 242, 249), 11 (p. 13), 12 (p. 104–105), 20 (pp. 326–327)]

Inferior colliculus. Along with the superior colliculus, the inferior colliculus forms the tectum, the roof of the midbrain. The inferior colliculus participates in auditory processing, receives input from cochlear nuclei, and relays impulses to the medial geniculate nucleus of the thalamus. The inferior colliculus is particularly important in auditory orienting behaviors.[2 (p 178), 12 (p 90), 20 (p 372)]

Inferior frontal gyrus.   This gyrus is located on the lateral, inferior part of the frontal lobe. It contains three divisions: orbital or anterior, opercular or posterior, and triangular (a middle wedge-shaped part). This gyrus, and particularly Broca's area of the dominant hemisphere (composed of opercular triangular divisions) is important for the production of spoken language.[6 (p. 18)]

Inferior frontal sulcus.   This structure divides the lateral surface of the frontal lobe.[12 (p. 219)]

Inferior nasal concha.   This structure is a thin bony plate that forms the lower part of the lateral wall of the nasal cavity.[14 (p. 348), 17 (p. 952)]

Inferior nasal meatus.   This is an opening in the cranium, which is overhung by the inferior nasal concha. It aids in warming and moistening inspired air.[4 (p. 313–314), 26 (p. 920)]

Inferior oblique muscle.   This muscle arises from the maxilla in the orbital floor and passes laterally and posteriorly below the inferior rectus muscle to insert on the sclera in the posteroinferior lateral orbit. It is innervated by the oculomotor nerve (III). The inferior oblique muscle serves to elevate the medially rotated eye and to abduct and rotate the eye laterally.[9 (pp. 715–717)]

Inferior olivary nucleus.   This nucleus receives afferents from the ipsilateral red nucleus, bilateral cortical areas (especially motor cortex), the cerebellar deep nuclei, and ascending spino-olivary fibers. The olivary complex gives rise to the climbing fiber system, which crosses the midline and ascends through the inferior cerebellar peduncle to all areas of the contralateral cerebellar hemisphere. It is involved in adaptive motor behavior allowing for the ability to modify motor responses to changing conditions.[1 (pp. 363–366), 6 (pp. 349–350)]

Inferior parietal lobule.   This lobule forms the posterior lateral portion of the parietal lobe. This region is involved in the integration of visual, auditory, and somatosensory functions, especially as related to written language.[3 (p. 409), 6 (p. 20), 14 (p. 848)]

Inferior rectus muscle.   This muscle is one of the four rectus muscles: superior, inferior, medial, and lateral, all of which arise from a common tendinous ring that surrounds the optic canal. The inferior rectus muscle passes anteriorly and inferiorly to attach to the eyeball posterior to the sclerocorneal junction. It is innervated by the oculomotor nerve (III) and serves to depress, adduct, and laterally rotate the eye.[9 (pp. 715–717)]

Inferior temporal gyrus.   The inferior temporal gyrus is located on the lateral and inferior surface of the brain and is separated from the middle temporal gyrus by the inferior temporal sulcus. This sulcus may be discontinuous and difficult to identify. The inferior temporal gyrus receives corticocortical projections for the analysis of the form and color of visual stimuli.[2 (pp. 154–157), 12 (p. 219)]

Infundibular recess.   This recess is one of two CSF-filled recesses in the floor of the third ventricle located on the medial hypothalamus. The second is the supraoptic recess located anteriorly and superiorly to the infundibular recess.[2 (p. 350)]

Infundibulum (pituitary stalk, hypophyseal stalk).   This structure connects the pituitary gland to the hypothalamus; it arises from the median eminence and is located between the optic chiasm and the mamillary bodies.[2 (p 355), 12 (p 196), 15 (p 739)]

Insular cortex (island of Reil).   This is an area of the cerebral cortex buried deep within the lateral (sylvian) sulcus. It is associated with visceral functions, and anteriorly it contains the cortical gustatory (taste) area. The areas covering the insula are referred to as the frontal, parietal, and temporal opercula.[2 (p. 196), 12 (p. 209), 19 (p. 294)]

Interhemispheric (longitudinal) fissure.   This fissure separates the cerebral hemispheres.[12 (p. 218), 19 (p. 257)]

Internal auditory canal.   The internal auditory canal is located in the petrous portion of the temporal bone anterior and superior to the jugular foramen and separated from the internal ear by a perforated bony plate. The facial nerve (VII), the auditory nerve (VIII), the nervous intermedius, and the labyrinthine vessels pass through this canal. [9] (p. 681)

Internal capsule-anterior limb.   This structure is a massive bundle of nerve fibers serving to interconnect subcortical nuclei with the cerebral cortex. It contains predominantly frontopontine and thalamocortical fibers to the frontal lobe. The distal radiating projection fibers to the cortex are referred to as the corona radiata. [7] (p. 12), [11] (p. 249), [16] (p. 538)

Internal capsule-genu.   This structure is located between the anterior and posterior limbs of the internal capsule. It contains descending corticobulbar and corticoreticular connection fibers. [7] (p. 12), [11] (p. 249), [16] (p. 538)

Internal capsule-posterior limb.   This structure contains fibers of general sensation. Corticospinal fibers that descend through this region are somatotopically organized with upper limb most rostral and lower limb caudal. (This is probably less precise than often depicted.) The most posterior nerve fibers radiate toward the calcarine sulcus and form the optic radiation. [7] (p. 12), [11] (p. 249), [16] (p. 538)

Internal carotid artery.   This artery arises from the common carotid artery. It supplies the eyes and associated tissues, pituitary gland, and anterior portions of the brain. Its chief branches are the anterior and middle cerebral arteries. [4] (p. 686)

Internal cerebral veins.   These vessels are paired veins formed from the thalamostriate and the choroid veins. They travel posteriorly with the tela choroidea of the third ventricle, joining beneath the splenium of the corpus callosum to form the great cerebral vein (vein of Galen). [11] (p. 455)

Internal jugular vein.   This vein originates as a dilation (superior bulb) below the posterior floor of the tympanic cavity, at the base of the skull in the jugular foramen. It is a direct continuation of the sigmoid sinus. The internal jugular vein serves as the primary venous drainage of the brain, face, and neck. [4] (p. 741), [8] (pp. 435–438)

Internal occipital crest and protuberance.   This structure forms a midline bony ridge that extends superiorly from the foramen magnum. It divides the posterior cranial fossa into two cerebellar fossae for the cerebellar hemispheres. This crest ends superiorly in an irregular elevation (referred to as the internal occipital protuberance) located at the level of the external occipital protuberance. [9] (p. 679)

Interpeduncular cistern.   This cistern is formed by an enlargement of the subarachnoid space on the anterior brainstem between the cerebral peduncles. It is filled with CSF. [7] (p. 69), [11] (p. 443)

Interpeduncular fossa.   This fossa is a subarachnoid space that lies between the cerebral peduncles on the ventral side of the brain, just posterior to the dorsum sella. Passing through this space are the oculomotor nerves, basilar artery, posterior communicating arteries, anterior choroidal arteries, superior cerebellar arteries, and the posterior cerebral arteries. The crural cisterns are lateral extensions of the interpeduncular cistern around the cerebral peduncles. [10] (pp. 116–117)

Jugular foramen.   This foramen is formed by the jugular fossa and the jugular notch of the occipital bone. It is a large, irregular cavity located at the posterior margin of the petro-occipital fissure directed forward, downward, and lateral. The jugular foramen is frequently larger on the right side. Passing through this foramen are the inferior petrosal sinus anteriorly; the glossopharyngeal, vagus, and accessory nerves intermediately; and the internal jugular vein posteriorly. [4] (pp. 307, 312, 329)

Lacrimal gland (sac).   Located in the superolateral orbit, this almond-shaped gland produces lacrimal fluid (tears) that moisten the cornea and wash away foreign material that may irritate the surface of the eye. [9] (pp. 711–712)

Lamina terminalis.   The lamina terminalis is the location of the anterior closure of the neural tube. This structure provides input to the hypothalamus regarding blood volume and blood pressure control.[2] (pp. 36, 356), [12] (pp. 196–197)

Lateral dorsal nucleus.   This nucleus, along with the anterior nuclear group (anterior ventral, anterior medial, and anterior dorsal), forms the major relay nuclei for the limbic system circuits. It has reciprocal connections with the cingulate gyrus and posterior parietal association areas.[1] (p. 444)

Lateral geniculate body (nucleus).   This is the principal thalamic relay nucleus for the visual system. It is a highly laminated structure with magnicellular and parvicellular divisions. There are two magnicellular layers (1 and 2), which receive input from contralateral and ipsilateral retinal ganglion cells (Y-type), respectively. Parvicellular layers 4 and 6 receive retinal ganglion cell input (X-type) from the contralateral retina, whereas layers 3 and 5 receive input from the ipsilateral retina. These connections are such that each lateral geniculate has a complete representation of the contralateral visual hemifield. Geniculate cells project to the primary visual cortex (striate cortex) located along the calcarine sulcus, in an orderly retinotopic fashion. It is noteworthy that the lateral geniculate actually receives more corticothalamic projections back from the cortex than it receives from the retina. This feedback network is believed to assist in regulating the flow of information to the primary visual cortex. In addition, such cortical back-projections may have a role in arousal and in regulating levels of visual attention.[1] (p 444), [2] (pp 154–160), [6] (p 288)

Lateral lemniscus.   This pathway consists of ascending fibers from the superior olivary complex and the cochlear nuclei that terminate in the inferior colliculus. This pathway transmits auditory information.[1] (p. 264), [3] (p. 199)

Lateral orbital gyrus of frontal lobe (gyrus rectus, straight gyrus).   This gyrus, part of the inferior frontal lobe, is located anteriorly and medial to the olfactory sulcus. Along with the remainder of the prefrontal cortex, it may be involved in higher cognitive processes relat-

ed to personality, insight, and foresight.[6] (pp. 18–20), [22] (p. 104)

Lateral posterior nucleus.   This is the largest nucleus in the lateral division of the lateral thalamic group. Along with the pulvinar and dorsolateral nucleus, this is one of the multimodal nuclei of the thalamus. It demonstrates extensive reciprocal connections with association areas of the parietal lobe.[1] (pp. 436–438), [22] (pp. 91–92)

Lateral rectus muscle.   This is one of the four rectus muscles: superior, inferior, medial, and lateral. All of these muscles arise from a common tendinous ring that surrounds the optic canal. It serves to rotate the eye so that the cornea is directed lateral. It is innervated by the abducens (VI) nerve.[9] (p. 715), [25] (p. 189)

Lateral spinothalamic tract.   This ascending pathway carries pain and temperature information from the contralateral side of the body to the thalamus.[2] (p. 125), [3] (p. 193)

Lateral ventricle.   This is an ependymal-lined C-shaped cavity of each hemisphere filled with CSF. The central lateral ventricle of the parietal lobe has horns extending into the frontal, occipital, and temporal lobes. CSF is formed by the choroid plexus located within the ventricle.[11] (p 183), [12] (pp. 253–256)

Lens.   This structure delineates the anterior chamber from the vitreous body and completes the refraction of entering light.[24] (p.p 283–287)

Lentiform nucleus.   This nucleus together with the caudate nucleus forms the corpus striatum, the major receiving station for the basal ganglia. It receives input from all regions of the cerebral cortex, some thalamic nuclei, the substantia nigra, and several brainstem nuclei. The lentiform nucleus is divided into the putamen and the globus pallidus, which project back to other basal ganglia nuclei, and the anterior and lateral nuclei of the thalamus. Like other basal ganglia nuclei, it is intimately involved in the modulation of motor function.[1] (p. 336), [12] (p. 207)

Lesser wing of the sphenoid bone.   Along with the orbital plates of the frontal bone, the lesser wing forms the majority of the floor of the posterior aspect of the anterior cranial fossa. The lesser wings of the sphenoid bone have sharp sphenoidal ridges where this bone projects into the anterior sylvian fissure. The lesser wings end medially at the anterior clinoid processes that serve as points of attachment for the tentorium cerebelli.[9] (p. 676)

Lingual gyrus (medial occipitotemporal gyrus). This gyrus is located on the inferior surface of the occipital lobe immediately posterior to the parahippocampal gyrus and is part of the visual cortex.[6] (pp. 21–22), [12] (pp. 221–223)

Lobule of the ear. Inferior margin of the external ear, the lobule is composed of fibrous and adipose tissue, providing for a soft compliant structure as compared to the more firm, elastic superior external ear.[4] (p. 1191)

Longus capitis muscle. This is one of the four anterior vertebral muscles (the others being longus colli, rectus capitis anterior, and rectus capitis lateralis). The longus capitis muscle serves to flex the head. It is innervated by the first, second, and third cervical spinal nerves.[4] (p. 541), [8] (p. 211)

Mamillary body. The mamillary bodies are found at the posterior extent of the hypothalamus and are an important part of the limbic system. They receive hippocampal input by way of the fornix. They project to the anterior nuclei of the dorsal thalamus and the midbrain tegmentum via mamillothalamic tract and mamillotegmental fasciculus, respectively. These structures are involved in limbic functions, including memory, emotion, and motivational behaviors.[1] (p. 386), [2] (pp. 367–368, 381, 392)

Mandible. This structure is comprised of two vertical rami and a horizontal horseshoe-shaped body. The mandible is the largest and strongest bone of the face. It serves as an attachment for muscles of mastication.[8] (p. 123), [17] (p. 815)

Massa intermedia (interthalamic adhesion). This structure is a midline nucleus of the thalamus. It joins the two thalami medially on an anatomic basis, but does not contain direct fiber connections across the midline.[1] (pp. 151, 433)

Masseter muscle. One of the four pairs of muscles of mastication used in biting and chewing

(the other three being temporalis, medial pterygoid, and lateral pterygoid), the masseter muscle raises the mandible to close the jaw.[4] (p. 534)

Mastoid process. This is a thick cone-shaped projection off the lower mastoid portion of the temporal bone lying behind and below the external auditory meatus. It contains air cells (sinuses) and serves as the attachment for the sternocleidomastoid, splenius capitis, and longus capitis muscles laterally. Medially, the mastoid notch provides attachment for the posterior belly of the digastric muscle.[4] (pp. 307, 328), [8] (p. 121)

Maxilla. This structure consists of a body and four processes: zygomatic, frontal, alveolar, and palatine. It forms the upper jaw, most of the roof of the mouth, and the floor and the lateral walls of the nasal cavity, as well as the floor of the orbit.[4] (pp. 338–340)

Maxillary sinus. Located in the maxilla, this sinus is lined with mucoperiosteum and filled with air. It acts as a resonator to the voice.[23] (pp. 734–736)

Meckel's cave (trigeminal cave). This cavity contains the proximal trigeminal ganglion and the roots of the trigeminal nerve. It is an extension of the subarachnoid space anteriorly and laterally from the lower layer of the tentorium, below the superior petrosal sinus, and near the apex of the petrous temporal bone.[4] (p. 1045), [12] (p. 382)

Medial geniculate body (nucleus). The medial geniculate nucleus is the auditory relay nucleus of the thalamus. It receives its dominant input from the inferior colliculus and it projects to the primary auditory cortex of the superior temporal gyrus. Both its input and output connections demonstrate an orderly tonotopic organization.[1] (p. 444), [3] (p. 193), [12] (p. 236), [15] (p. 181)

Medial longitudinal fasciculus. This is a brainstem pathway that contains ascending and descending fibers that interconnect the vestibular nuclei with nuclei involved in the control of eye movements and the integration of eye, head, and neck movements.[2] (p. 173)

Medial lemniscus. The medial lemniscus contains ascending fibers from the dorsal column nuclei to the thalamus. As such, the medial lemniscus carries somatosensory information related to touch and proprioception. Unilateral lesions of the medial lemniscus cause contralateral deficits because the ascending fibers from the dorsal column nuclei decussate (as internal arcuate fibers) prior to entering the lemniscus.[1] (pp. 203–206), [18] (p. 740)

Medial rectus muscle.   One of the four rectus muscles: superior, inferior, medial, and lateral, all of which arise from a common tendinous ring that surrounds the optic canal. This muscle rotates the eye so that the cornea is directed medially (adduction). It is innervated by the oculomotor (III) nerve.[9] (p. 715), [25] (p. 189)

Median eminence.   Together with the pituitary, the median eminence forms the neurohypophysis. It is located at the junction of the hypothalamus and pituitary stalk. The median eminence is a highly vascularized region whose capillaries lack a blood–brain barrier. Many hypothalamic neurons release peptide neurohormones and regulatory factors into the hypothalamo-hypophysial portal circulation, through which they influence hormone release by the anterior pituitary.[1] (p. 176), [2] (p. 365), [3] (pp. 421–424)

Medulla oblongata (myelencephalon or medulla).   The medulla oblongata is one of the three parts of the brainstem, the other two being the pons and midbrain. It serves to connect the spinal cord and the brain and contains centers for autonomic function such as digestion, breathing, blood pressure, and heart rate. The medulla also contains the pyramidal decussation inferiorly where most of the corticospinal tract crosses the midline, allowing for contralateral corticomotor control. The nuclei for cranial nerves VIII, IX, X, XI, XII, and parts of V, as well as the inferior olivary complex are located in the medulla.[1] (pp. 15, 132–133), [2] (p. 9), [13] (p. 7), [15] (p. 9)

Midbrain (mesencephalon).   The midbrain is the smallest of the three parts of the brainstem, the other two being the pons and the medulla oblongata. Ventrally the midbrain contains the tegmentum, which houses the red nucleus, and the substantia nigra (important motor nuclei). The tectum, which contains the inferior and superior colliculi, is located at the dorsal surface of the midbrain. The tectum is involved in auditory and visual processing, especially in relation to control of eye movements and orienting behaviors.[15] (p. 276)

Middle cerebellar peduncle.   This structure connects the cerebellum to the pons. It contains primarily afferent axons relaying input from the contralateral cerebral cortex through the pontine nuclei to the lateral lobe of the cerebellum.[2] (pp. 242, 249), [11] (p. 13), [12] (pp. 104–105)

Middle cerebral artery.   This artery is a branch of the internal carotid artery that provides vascular supply to the region of the insular cortex and the lateral surface of the hemisphere.[1] (p. 186), [10] (pp. 207–211)

Middle frontal gyrus.   This gyrus participates with the primary motor cortex in the control and initiation of voluntary movements. It is part of the prefrontal cortex and it supports higher cognitive functions related to personality, insight, and foresight.[6] (p. 18)

Middle nasal concha.   This structure is the lower of two bony plates that project from the ethmoid bone. A mucosal-covered surface, it separates the superior and middle nasal meatus, and forms the boundary of the air passageway or meatus. [14] (p. 348), [17] (p. 952)

Middle nasal meatus.   This structure is part of the nasal cavity bounded superiorly by the middle nasal concha and inferiorly by the inferior nasal concha. It aids in warming and moistening inspired air.[4] (pp. 313–314), [14] (p. 920)

Middle temporal gyrus.   This gyrus is one of the three principal gyri that run parallel to the sylvian fissure located on the lateral surface of the brain. This region includes multimodal association areas believed to be involved in perceptual and mnemonic integration.[22] (p. 107)

Middle temporal sulcus.   The middle temporal sulcus divides the middle and inferior temporal gyri.[1] (p. 161)

Nasal bone.   This is one of the bones of the face. The right and left nasal bones articulate with each other at the internasal suture to form the bridge of the nose.[9] (p. 651)

Nasal cavity. This cavity is divided into right and left halves by the nasal septum. The nasal cavity extends from the nostrils in front to the conchae behind where the nose opens into the nasopharynx. It aids in warming and moistening inspired air.[4] (p. 1142)

Nasal septum. The nasal septum is a partition composed of cartilaginous, membranous, and bony parts. It separates the right and left nasal fossae (cavities).[14] (p. 1402)

Nasolacrimal canal. This canal is formed by the inferior nasal concha, the lacrimal bone, and the lacrimal sulcus of the maxilla. It contains the nasolacrimal duct.[14] (p. 251)

Nasopharynx. This structure is one of the three parts of the pharynx (the other two being the oral and the laryngeal). It extends from the posterior nasal cavity to the soft palate. It communicates anteriorly with the nasal cavities and laterally with the middle ear through the eustachian (auditory) tubes. Posterior to the eustachian tube openings is a raised area called the torus tubarius. Posteriorly, the nasopharynx approximates the distance from the middle of the clivus to the body of the second cervical vertebrae. Its primary purpose is to assist in respiration.[8] (pp. 468, 469), [24] (p. 462)

Nucleus ambiguus. This nucleus contains motor neurons with fibers in the glossopharyngeal (IX), vagus (X), and spinal accessory (XI) nerves for innervation of muscles of the palate, pharynx, and larynx. It is one of four cranial nerve nuclei within the brainstem motor nuclear column, which is comprised of: (1) trigeminal motor nucleus; (2) facial motor nucleus; (3) nucleus ambiguus; and (4) accessory nucleus.[2] (pp. 322–333)

Neurohypophysis (posterior lobe of the pituitary gland). Composed of the median eminence, infundibular stalk, and the posterior lobe of the pituitary gland, the neurohypophysis mediates regulatory functions of the nervous system. It is the only mammalian example of a neurohemal organ consisting of neurosecretory axons ending on capillary blood vessels. Phylogenetically, it is one of the oldest neuronal structures. It receives vaso-pressin-containing fibers from the supraoptic nucleus of the hypothalamus and oxytocin-containing fibers from the paraventricular nucleus of the hypothalamus. These hormones enter the bloodstream by way of the capillary bed throughout the neurohypophysis (primarily the posterior lobe of the pituitary gland).[12] (pp. 196, 201–203)

Occipital bone. A cuplike structure forming the inferior and anterior walls of the posterior fossa, the occipital bone is pierced centrally by the oval foramen magnum. Its basilar part is anterior to the foramen magnum, its squama is posterior, and on either side are the lateral portions. It supports the medulla oblongata and the lower part of the pons and gives attachment to the tentorium cerebelli. It contains the foramen for the hypoglossal nerve, passage of spinal cord, accessory nerves, vertebral arteries, and posterior spinal arteries.[4] (pp. 319–322)

Occipital lobe. This lobe contains the primary visual cortex and the visual association cortex involved in the higher order processing of visual information.[6] (pp. 21–22)

Occipital pole. The occipital pole is the most posterior aspect of the occipital cortex and is located posterior to the parietal occipital sulcus. This area may contain part of the primary visual cortex, which receives afferent fibers from the lateral geniculate body.[11] (pp. 236, 265)

Oculomotor nerve (cranial nerve III). This nerve innervates four of the six extraocular muscles: (1) superior rectus, which provides superior and medial eye deviation; (2) medial rectus, which provides medial deviation (adduction); (3) inferior rectus, which provides inferior and medial deviation; and (4) inferior oblique, which provides superior and lateral deviation. It also provides innervation for the levator palpebrae, which elevates the eyelid.[2] (pp. 322–333), [25] (p. 189)

Oculomotor nucleus. This is the first member of the general somatic motor column: oculomotor nucleus, trochlear nucleus, abducens nucleus, and hypoglossal nucleus. It contains the motor neurons projecting peripherally through the oculomotor nerve, which exits the ventral midbrain at the level of the cerebral peduncle.[2] (pp. 322–333)

Odontoid process (dens) of axis (C2). This strong toothlike structure projects upward from the body of the second cervical vertebrae and is the embryological body of the atlas. It is contained in the anterior compartment of the vertebral foramen of the atlas by the transverse ligament. This structure serves as the pivot around which the atlas rotates.[4] (pp. 273–274), [8] (pp. 129–130)

Olfactory bulb. These are a pair of laminar telencephalic expansions located within the cranial cavity just above the cribriform plate and receiving projections of the olfactory nerves. The central core of the olfactory bulbs projects posteriorly as the olfactory tract.[1] (p. 293)

Olfactory nerve (cranial nerve I). The fibers of the olfactory nerve consist of unmyelinated axons of olfactory neurosensory cells from the olfactory neuroepithelium covering the superior concha of the nasal cavity and the superior nasal septum. These axons form 18 to 20 nerve bundles that together make up the olfactory nerves passing through the cribriform plate to enter the olfactory bulbs. The olfactory nerve is the nerve of smell.[9] (p. 853)

Olfactory sulcus. Located deep to the olfactory bulbs and tracts, this sulcus forms the lateral margin of the gyrus rectus.[1] (p. 160)

Olfactory tract. This is a continuation of the central core of the olfactory bulbs projecting to the olfactory cortex of the brain in the region of the anterior perforated substance and the uncus.[1] (p. 294), [9] (p. 853)

Olive. This structure is a prominent oval swelling of the ventral medulla produced by the underlying inferior olivary complex. This complex is composed of three parts: inferior olivary nucleus, medial accessory olivary nucleus, and dorsal accessory olivary nucleus. The accessory olivary nuclei project to the cerebellar vermis and adjacent cortex and are concerned with the maintenance of equilibrium, posture, and locomotion. The inferior olivary nucleus projects to the cerebellum, cerebellar nuclei, red nucleus, periaqueductal gray,

and the cerebral cortex, providing efficiency of precise voluntary movements. The inferior olivary complex is involved in the coordination of learned movement.[12] (pp. 85–86, 96–99)

Optic canal. This canal is located in the anteromedial part of the middle cranial fossa and connects this space with the orbit. It is traversed by the optic nerve (cranial nerve II) and the ophthalmic arteries.[9] (p. 679)

Optic chiasm. This structure represents the convergence of the optic nerves forming a flattened bundle of fibers at the junction of the anterior wall and floor of the third ventricle. Fibers from the nasal region of each retina decussate at this location, entering the contralateral optic tract, while the lateral fibers pass directly to the ipsilateral optic tract.[2] (p. 143), [11] (p. 227)

Optic nerve (cranial nerve II). This nerve is the primary nerve of sight; it is composed of the axons of the ganglion cells of the retina. Most of the fibers originating from the nasal retina of each eye decussate at the optic chiasm and project to the contralateral geniculate nucleus. Most fibers from the temporal retinae project to the ipsilateral geniculate nucleus. Some optic nerve fibers project to the superior colliculi, several pretectal nuclei, and some subcortical nuclei located in the vicinity of the optic chiasm.[7] (pp. 221, 227)

Optic radiation. This pathway consists of the projection fibers from the lateral geniculate body (nucleus) that terminate in the primary visual cortex (V-1) of the occipital lobe. These fibers traverse the internal capsule and course around the lateral wall of the lateral ventricle toward the medial and posterior occipital cortex. The fibers representing the upper quadrant of the visual field travel anteriorly, laterally, and then posteriorly. As they near the anterior tip of the temporal horn, these fibers form a bundle known as Meyer's loop. The optic radiations maintain a precise visuotopic organization from the lateral geniculate body to the primary visual cortex.[1] (p. 240)

Optic recess. This is a pointed projection of the third ventricle located anterior and superior to the optic chiasm.[3] (p. 315)

Optic tract. The optic tract is that portion of the optic nerve located between the chiasm and lateral geniculate.[15] (p. 424), [19] (p. 399)

Orbital fat. The orbital fat provides cushioning and support for the eye; occupies the space within the orbit not occupied by the globe, nerves, muscles, and vessels; and is bounded anteriorly by the orbital septum and posteriorly by the orbital apex.[25] (p. 188)

Orbital gyrus. This gyrus is located on the ventral surface of the frontal lobe, lateral to the olfactory bulb and tract. It receives projection fibers from the mediodorsal nucleus of the thalamus and is essential for the conscious perception of odors. This gyrus is also involved in providing affective and emotional dimensions to olfaction.[1] (pp. 160, 296, 463)

Orbital sulcus. This sulcus forms the lateral margin of the lateral gyrus.[1] (pp. 159–161)

Oropharynx. This structure is one of the three parts of the pharynx, the other two being the nasal and the laryngeal. It extends from the soft palate to the hyoid bone and contains the palatine tonsils laterally. Posteriorly, the oropharynx approximates the distance from the body of the second cervical vertebrae to the middle of the third vertebral body. It receives food from the mouth and air from the nasopharynx.[4] (p. 1309), [8] (pp. 468–469)

Paracentral lobule. The paracentral lobule refers to the extensions of the precentral (motor) and postcentral (sensory) gyri onto the medial surface of the hemisphere.[6] (pp. 18–20)

Paracentral sulcus. Located immediately anterior to the paracentral lobule, the paracentral sulcus is a branch of the cingulate sulcus before it divides into the marginal and subparietal sulci.[12] (pp. 221–222)

Parahippocampal gyrus. The parahippocampal gyrus, located in the medial temporal lobe, contains the piriform cortex rostrally and entorhinal cortex caudally. It is an important part of the limbic system that is involved in olfactory and memory perceptions.[2] (pp. 200–202), [15] (pp. 306 307)

Paraventricular nucleus. This gyrus is located in the chiasmatic region. Its output fibers project down the infundibular stalk to the neurohypophysis. It is a prominent nucleus of the hypothalamus, which with the supraoptic nucleus of the hypothalamus has neurosecretory functions. It produces the neurohormones vasopressin and oxytocin. Vasopressin (antidiuretic hormone [ADH]) has multiple functions, including promotion of water reabsorption by the kidneys and elevation of blood pressure. Oxytocin functions to promote the ejection of milk from the mammary glands and stimulates uterine contractions.[1] (pp. 384–385), [2] (p. 354)

Parietal bone. With the frontal and parts of the temporal and sphenoid bones, the parietal bone forms the lateral aspect of the skull. It encloses and protects the brain.[9] (p. 641), [24] (p. 170)

Parietal lobe. This lobe is bounded anteriorly by the central sulcus, posteriorly by a line through the parieto-occipital sulcus, and inferiorly by a line extended from the posterior ramus of the sylvian fissure. The parietal lobe contains primary and higher order association somatosensory areas. The primary somatosensory cortex is located on the postcentral gyrus. The second somatosensory area is located at the inferior margin of the postcentral gyrus along the superior sylvian fissure. Involved in less discriminative and possible mnemonic functions, this area may extend onto the insular cortex. Additional association cortex is located primarily in the superior parietal lobule and in the precuneus. It is concerned with integrating information from the general senses and it allows for processing the significance of sensory data. Additional auditory and visual integration areas, as well as regions involved in spatial perception, are located in the parietal lobe.[9] (p. 693), [12] (pp. 232–235)

Parietal occipital sulcus. This sulcus separates the parietal and occipital lobes and meets with the calcarine sulcus.[11] (p. 233), [19] (p. 259)

Periaqueductal gray matter. These undifferentiated gray (cellular) areas form the walls or floor of the cerebral aqueduct. They play a role in endogenous pain suppression and contain high concentrations of opioid peptides (endorphins).[1] (p. 220), [2] (p. 68)

Pineal gland.   Along with the habenular nuclei and the stria medullaris, the pineal gland forms the epithalamus. The pineal gland is not directly photosensitive in humans, but it does receive light cycle information from the suprachiasmatic nucleus of the hypothalamus through sympathetic fibers from the superior cervical ganglia. The pineal is involved in the cyclic production of hormones such as melatonin. The pineal gland also contains biogenic amines and neuroactive peptides. It is associated with the mechanisms that regulate circadian rhythm.[1] (p. 149), [8] (pp. 435–438)

Pituitary fossa (hypophyseal fossa).   This fossa is one of the three parts of the sella turcica: (1) olive-shaped anterior swelling, the tuberculum sellae; (2) the seatlike depression, the pituitary fossa; and (3) the posterior dorsum sellae. It contains the pituitary gland.[9] (p. 676)

Pituitary gland (hypophysis).   It consists of an anterior lobe (adenohypophysis), a nonfunctional pars intermedia, and a posterior lobe (neurohypophysis). The anterior lobe produces numerous hormones, including growth hormone, thyroid-stimulating hormone, follicle-stimulating hormone, luteinizing hormone, ACTH, and prolactin. The posterior lobe is a neurohemal organ composed of neurosecretory axons ending on capillary blood vessels and contains vasopressin (ADH) and oxytocin, which are synthesized in the hypothalamus. The hypothalamus regulates nearly all organs of the body by means of the hypothalamo-hypophysial tract, pituitary hormones, and modulating actions of the autonomic nervous system.[1] (pp. 421–424), [2] (p. 350), [12] (pp. 201–203)

Pons.   The pons is one of the three parts of the brainstem. It connects the remaining two parts, which are the medulla oblongata and the midbrain. The pons contains neural circuits that transmit information between the spinal cord and higher brain regions. Along with the medulla and midbrain, the pons regulates levels of arousal through the central part of the brainstem (the reticular formation). Together with the medulla, pontine nuclei regulate blood pressure and respiration. Other pontine nuclei play a major role in motor function, serving to relay information between the cerebral cortex and the cerebellum.[2] (p. 9), [11] (p. 181)

Pontine cistern.   This is a CSF-filled space located between the pons and the upper clivus, joined laterally by the cerebellopontine angle cistern and superiorly by the interpeduncular cistern. It contains the trigeminal and abducens nerves, the basilar artery, and the anterior inferior cerebellar artery.[10] (pp. 115–116)

Postcentral gyrus.   This area of the cortex includes Brodmann's areas 1, 2, and 3, which are associated with processing somatosensory information. This gyrus lies posterior to the central sulcus and anterior to the postcentral sulcus in the parietal lobe. It is concerned with the processing of tactile and proprioceptive (sense of position) information. It receives input from the ventral posterior lateral and ventral posterior medial thalamic nuclei. This input shows a high degree of somatotopy in the form of an inverted homunculus, with information from the lower extremities projecting to the superomedial surface, and information from the face projecting to the inferolateral surface.[6] (pp. 18–20)

Postcentral sulcus.   This sulcus lies behind the postcentral gyrus in the parietal lobe.[6] (pp. 18–20)

Posterior cerebral artery.   This artery arises from the terminal branches of the basilar artery, usually bifurcating in the interpeduncular cistern. It supplies the inferior and medial surfaces of the parietal and temporal lobes.[1] (p. 186), [10] (pp. 248–251)

Posterior commissure.   This is a bundle of nerve fibers crossing the midline immediately above the cerebral aqueduct at the junction of the third ventricle. It is the attachment site for the inferior pineal stalk. It receives fibers from the superior colliculus, the pretectal area, the habenular nuclei, and the accessory oculomotor nuclei. Of particular import are decussating fibers from the pretectal nuclei to parasympathetic preganglionic neurons that mediate the pupillary light reflex.[11] (p. 246), [12] (p. 195)

Posterior communicating artery.   This artery

arises from the internal carotid artery and serves to join the internal carotid with the posterior cerebral artery.[1] (p. 179), [10] (p. 179)

Posterior horn of the lateral ventricle. This structure extends into the occipital lobe with the roof and lateral wall formed by the tapetum of the corpus callosum. It contains two medial wall elevations that are caused by the forceps major superiorly and by an inferior elevation resulting from the calcarine sulcus (referred to as the calcar avis).[11] (pp. 242, 260)

Precentral gyrus. This gyrus lies behind the precentral sulcus and anterior to the central sulcus in the parietal lobe. It is the location of primary motor cortex, Brodmann's area 4. It receives input from multiple cortical areas and also dorsal thalamic nuclei, which relay information from the somatosensory system, vestibular system, the cerebellum, and the basal ganglia. It gives rise to descending corticospinal, corticostriatal, corticorubral, and corticothalamic projections that influence motor activity. As with the postcentral gyrus, the precentral gyrus shows somatotopic organization in the form of an inverted homunculus, with information from the lower extremities projecting to the superomedial surface, and information from the face projecting to the inferolateral surface.[1] (pp. 157, 326–327)

Precentral sulcus. This sulcus is located anterior to the precentral gyrus and divides the precentral gyrus from the remainder of the frontal lobe.[6] (pp. 18–20)

Precuneus (quadrate lobe). The precuneus is a square-shaped medial convolution of the parietal lobe. Posteriorly, it extends to the parieto-occipital sulcus and anteriorly it extends to the paracentral lobule. Superiorly, the precuneus is involved in complex sensory appreciation. Medially, it is involved in language comprehension in the dominant hemisphere and may be involved in complex aspects of orientation to time and space.[3] (p. 404), [6] (pp. 18–20), [14] (p. 1249)

Pretectal area. Composed of four nuclei located immediately in front of the lateral margin of the superior colliculus, the pretectal area receives projections from the retina via the optic tract and superior brachium. Additional afferents come from the superior colliculi and visual cortex. Its dominant efferent connections are to the Edinger-Westphal nucleus, which gives rise to parasympathetic innervation to the eye and preganglionic fibers to the ciliary ganglion, all of which travel as part of the oculomotor nerve. Additional efferents project to the accessory oculomotor nuclei. The pretectal area is involved in a reflex pathway for pupillary light response and cortical control of eye movement.[1] (p. 411), [12] (p. 112)

Pterygopalatine fossa. This is a pyramidal-shaped space located inferior to the apex of the orbit with the superior margin opening into the inferior orbital fissure. Laterally, it opens into the infratemporal fossa, and is closed inferiorly except for the palatine foramina. Posterosuperiorly, this fossa communicates with the middle cranial fossa through the foramen rotundum. The pterygopalatine fossa contains the pterygopalatine ganglion, the terminal branches of the maxillary artery, and the second division of the trigeminal nerve (cranial nerve V[2], maxillary nerve).[9] (p. 752)

Pulvinar nucleus. Along with the posterolateral and dorsolateral nuclei, the pulvinar nucleus forms the multimodal functional division of the thalamic nuclei. These multimodal nuclei are connected with association areas of the parietal lobe. The pulvinar may play an important role in modulation of visual attention.[3] (pp. 144–145), [22] (pp. 90–92)

Putamen. Together with the globus pallidus, the putamen forms the lenticular nucleus. The putamen and the caudate nucleus are often collectively referred to as the neostriatum. The putamen receives input from the motor and somatosensory areas of the cortex and projects by way of the globus pallidus and the thalamus to the supplementary motor area. It is centrally involved in motor function.[6] (p. 304), [7] (p. 11)

Pyramid. Located on the ventral medulla, the pyramids contain descending motor fibers of the lateral and ventral corticospinal tracts as well as the corticobulbar tracts.[2] (p. 229)

Pyramidal (corticospinal) tract. The pyramidal tract originates primarily in the motor cortex (with additional fibers from primary somatosensory cortex and association sensorimotor areas) and projects to lower motor neurons of the spinal cord. These descending fibers from the motor cortex cross the midline at the medullary level, so that the motor cortex of one hemisphere controls voluntary motor activity on the opposite side of the body.[2] (pp. 208–210), [3] (p. 193), [12] (p. 148)

Pyramidal decussation.   The pyramidal decussation is located at the junction of the spinal cord and medulla, where approximately 85% of the pyramidal fibers cross to enter the opposite lateral corticospinal tract, allowing one side of the brain to control the opposite side of the body. The remaining 15% of the uncrossed fibers enter the ventral corticospinal tract.[12] (p. 336)

Quadrigeminal plate cistern (retropulvinar cistern).   This cistern is an enlarged subarachnoid space containing CSF and located posterior to the superior and inferior colliculi. It merges on either side with the ambient cisterns and the wings of the ambient cisterns. It communicates posteriorly with the superior cerebellar cistern and anteriorly with the suprapineal recess of the third ventricle. The pineal body is contained in the anterior part of this cistern.[10] (pp. 120–121)

Raphe nuclei (paramedian raphe).   Located within the midline of the brainstem, cells of the raphe nuclei are the dominant source of ascending and descending serotonergic fibers to the cerebral cortex and spinal cord, respectively. The cells of the raphe form in an irregular but contiguous column interspersed among bundles of decussating myelinated axons. The raphe nuclei modulate the general behavioral state, perception of pain, and the sleep-wake cycle.[1] (p. 220), [12] (p. 149), [13] (p. 231)

Rectus capitis posterior major muscle.   This muscle is one of the suboccipital muscles originating on the spinous process of the axis and inserting on the occipital bone. It serves to extend and rotate the head.[4] (pp. 546–547), [8] (pp. 211, 255–268)

Rectus capitis posterior minor muscle.   This muscle is one of the suboccipital muscles originating on the posterior arch of the atlas and inserting on the occipital bone. It serves to extend the head.[4] (pp. 546–547), [8] (pp. 211, 255–268)

Red nucleus.   The red nucleus is part of the tegmentum and relays impulses from the cerebral and cerebellar cortex to the spinal cord with feedback to the cerebellum. The red nucleus receives input from ipsilateral cerebral cortex and contralateral deep cerebellar nuclei. It gives rise to reciprocal connections to the cerebellar nuclei, the contralateral rubrospinal tract, and rubrobulbar tract. Motor disturbances attributed to destruction of the red nucleus include contralateral tremor, ataxia, and choreiform movements, a condition known as the syndrome of Benedikt.[1] (p. 353), [2] (pp. 225–226, 250), [16] (pp. 435–436)

Reticular formation.   The reticular formation occupies the central core of the brainstem and receives information from most of the sensory systems. Having direct and indirect efferent connections to all levels of the central nervous system, it is involved in the modulation of attentional state (sleep and arousal), motor functions, and assorted visceral activities.[2] (p. 229), [12] (p. 148)

Rostrum of corpus callosum.   The rostrum refers to the anteroinferior aspect of the corpus callosum. It is continuous with the genu above and the lamina terminalis below and forms the anterior wall of the third ventricle. The rostrum contains interhemispheric connections between prefrontal regions.[12] (pp. 246, 248)

Sclera.   The sclera is continuous with the dura of the optic nerve and the dural covering of the brain. This covering forms the "white" of the eye.[9] (pp. 705–708)

Semicircular canals.   Made up of anterior, posterior, and lateral canals, the fluid-filled semicircular canals communicate with the bony labyrinth and are positioned at right angles to each other. These canals support vestibular functions related to maintenance of balance and equilibrium.[6] (pp. 210–215), [9] (pp. 774–776)

Semispinalis capitis muscle.   This muscle is

one of the posterior muscles of the head and neck arising from the transverse processes of the seventh cervical and the superior six or seven thoracic vertebrae inserting on the medial occipital bone. It serves to extend and rotate the head.[4] (p. 545), [8] (pp. 211, 255–268)

Septal nuclei.   Consisting of separate medial and lateral subdivisions, the septal nuclei are continuous with the gray matter on the medial surface of the cerebral hemisphere, just rostral to the lamina terminalis. The septal nuclei have extensive reciprocal connections with the hippocampus, hypothalamus, and habenula. Lesions of the septal nuclei can produce rage behavior, whereas electrical stimulation of this area is associated with "pleasure" sensations.[1] (pp. 493–494), [2] (pp. 385–386)

Septum pellucidum.   This structure forms the medial wall of the body and anterior horns of the lateral ventricle. It is continuous inferiorly with the septal nuclei and actually contains a small portion of the septal nuclei along with white matter fibers. This double-membrane, connective tissue structure is covered on either side by ependyma and contains a slitlike cavity, the cavum septum pellucidum.[2] (p. 384), [12] (pp. 249–250), [19] (p. 373)

Septum of the tongue.   The septum is the vertical median fibrous part of the tongue that divides it into halves.[9] (p. 746), [14] (p. 1402)

Sigmoid venous sinus.   The sigmoid, an S-shaped dural sinus, receives most of the blood supply from the dural venous sinuses terminating in the internal jugular veins at the level of the jugular foramen.[1] (pp. 187–188), [17] (p. 867)

Soft palate.   Along with the hard palate, the soft palate forms the roof of the mouth. It is a flexible, musculomembranous curtain lying posterior to the hard palate and extending downward and backward between the oral and nasal parts of the pharynx, with a small conical process (uvula) hanging from the middle of the lower margin. It plays an important role in swallowing, speech, and blowing air out through the mouth while preventing release through the nose.[4] (pp. 1270,1313), [8] (p. 467)

Sphenoid bone.   This bone is located anterior to the temporal bone and has a wedge shape. It articulates with eight bones of the skull: frontal, parietal, temporal, occipital, vomer, zygomatic, palatine, and ethmoid. It consists of a body as well as greater and lesser wings that spread out laterally from the body. The superior surface of the body is shaped like a Turkish saddle and is referred to as the sella turcica. The sella turcica contains the pituitary gland.[9] (p. 645)

Sphenoid sinus.   This sinus is one of the paranasal sinuses. It is an air-filled cavity located in the sphenoid bone, closely associated with the optic nerves and optic chiasm, pituitary gland, internal carotid artery, and cavernous sinuses. It acts as a resonator to the voice.[23] (p. 734–736)

Spinal cord.   The spinal cord is an elongated cylindrical part of the central nervous system extending from the level of the atlas to approximately the level of the first and second lumbar vertebrae. It measures 6 to 12 mm in width and 42 cm in length in the adult female and 45 cm in the adult male. It weighs approximately 30 g and represents about 2% of the central nervous system. This structure innervates the motor and sensory areas of the entire body with the exception of those innervated by the cranial nerves.[1] (p. 117), [4] (p. 864)

Splenium of corpus callosum.   The splenium is an enlargement of the corpus callosum, posteriorly connecting the occipital lobes and forming the forceps occipitalis (forceps major).[11] (pp. 244–245), [12] (p. 248), [19] (p. 269)

Splenius capitis muscle.   This is one of the posterior muscles of the head and neck. It originates with the ligamentum nuchae and the spinous processes of the seventh cervical and superior three thoracic vertebrae. It inserts on the occipital and mastoid processes of the temporal bone. It serves to extend, rotate, and laterally flex the neck.[4] (p. 543), [8] (pp. 211, 255–268)

Squamous portion of the occipital bone.   This structure is one of four parts of the occipital bone: squamous, basilar, and two condylar (lateral) parts. The four parts are developmentally separate and unite around the foramen magnum at approximately 6 years of age. The internal squamous part is divided into four fossae. The two superior fossae contain the occipital poles, and the inferior two (referred to as the cerebellar fossae) contain the cerebellar hemispheres. The squamous portion provides protection for the underlying brain.[9] (p. 650)

Sternocleidomastoid muscle. This is one of two lateral cervical muscles, the other being the trapezius. It consists of two heads, one on the clavicle and the other on the manubrium of the sternum, with insertion on the mastoid process of the temporal bone. The unilateral action of this muscle draws the head to the side, and bilateral contraction of the muscle serves to flex the vertebral column, the head, and elevate the chin. It is also involved in head rotation.[4] (pp. 538–539), [8] (pp. 208, 255–268)

Straight venous sinus. This is one of the dural sinuses providing cerebral venous drainage. It forms at the junction of the falx and the tentorium by union of the inferior sagittal sinus and the great cerebral vein of Galen. It terminates more commonly to the left, forming the transverse sinus.[7] (p. 61), [15] (pp. 440–441)

Stria terminalis. The stria terminalis is a fiber pathway that connects the amygdala to the septal nuclei. Extending along the inner curvature of the caudate nucleus, this projection is an important component of the limbic system, especially in its role as a mediator of emotion.[1] (p. 493)

Substantia nigra. The substantia nigra is a large midbrain nucleus located between the tegmentum and basis pedunculi. It is an important component of the basal ganglia with connections to the ventral medial nucleus of the thalamus, amygdaloid body, putamen, caudate, and superior colliculus. The pars compacta region contains dopaminergic neurons that project to and regulate neostriatal motor functions. These cells degenerate in Parkinson's disease, and their loss causes a resting tremor and other motor problems.[12] (pp. 114–115), [20] (pp. 276–277)

Subthalamic nucleus (nucleus of Luys). Located next to the internal capsule, the subthalamic nucleus is a motor nucleus of the basal ganglia with reciprocal connections to the globus pallidus (through the subthalamic fasciculus which crosses the internal capsule). The subthalamus is formed of the subthalamic nucleus, sensory fasciculi, extensions of midbrain nuclei, bundles of fibers from cerebellar nuclei, and the globus pallidus. A lesion of the subthalamic nucleus results in contralateral hemiballismus.[12] (pp. 193–194)

Subthalamus. The subthalamus contains the subthalamic nucleus, extensions of midbrain nuclei, bundles of fibers from cerebellar nuclei, the globus pallidus, and sensory fasciculi. It is primarily involved in motor function. This part of the brain is also important in the regulation of drinking behaviors.[1] (pp. 149–150), [12] (pp. 193–194)

Superior cerebellar cistern. The superior cerebellar cistern is not a true cistern, but rather a broad flat space between the undersurface of the tentorium and the upper surface of the cerebellum. This space communicates with the quadrigeminal cistern anteromedially, the ambient cisterns anterolaterally, and the general subarachnoid spaces around the cerebellum peripherally. This space does not normally contain anatomically important structures.[10] (p. 120)

Superior cerebellar peduncle. This structure connects the cerebellum to the midbrain. It carries primarily cerebellar efferent projections that originate in cerebellar nuclei and enter the brainstem just caudal to the inferior colliculus. The peduncle also contains afferent projections of the rubrocerebellar tract, tectocerebellar tract, and the anterior spinocerebellar tract, all of which project the cerebellar cortex.[2] (pp. 242, 249), [11] (p. 13), [12] (pp. 104–105), [20] (p. 326)

Superior colliculus. The superior colliculus is located posterior and medial to the lateral geniculate body (nucleus) in the roof (tectum) of the midbrain. It represents a reflex center for somatic motor reflexes in response to visual stimuli and it receives visual signals directly from the retina or indirectly from the visual cortex. The retinotectal projections create a visuotopic map of each contralateral visual hemifield in each superior colliculus. This structure is essential for rapid eye movements.

Damage to the superior colliculus causes a loss of conjugate upward eye movement (Parinaud's syndrome).[1] (pp. 245–246, 412)

Superior frontal gyrus. This gyrus is part of the frontal lobe that participates with the primary motor cortex in the control and initiation of voluntary movements. It is part of the prefrontal cortex involved in higher cognitive functions related to personality, insight awareness, and judgment.[6] (pp. 18–20), [18] (p. 674), [19] (p. 260)

Superior frontal sulcus. This sulcus separates the superior frontal gyrus from the middle frontal gyrus.[12] (p. 219)

Superior medullary velum. This is a thin structure extending between the superior cerebellar peduncles and forming part of the roof of the fourth ventricle.[1] (pp. 136–137)

Superior muscle bundle. This muscle bundle contains the superior rectus (providing for superior and medial orbit deviation, with third nerve innervation) and the superior oblique muscles (providing for inferior and lateral orbit deviation, with fourth nerve innervation).[25] (p. 189)

Superior nasal concha. This structure is the upper of two bony plates that project from the ethmoid bone. It forms the upper boundary of the superior meatus.[14] (p. 348), [17] (p. 952)

Superior nasal meatus. This structure is the shortest and most shallow of the nasal meatuses. It communicates with the posterior ethmoidal air cells and serves to warm and moisturize inspired air.[4] (pp. 313–314), [14] (p. 920)

Superior oblique muscle. This muscle originates from the body of the sphenoid bone and passes anterosuperiorly and medially to the superior and medial rectus muscles, ending in a round tendon running through a loop (pulley) called the trochlea, which is attached to the superior medial angle of the orbit. From the trochlea, the tendon turns posterolaterally for insertion into the sclera at the posterosuperior margin of the lateral orbit. It is innervated by cranial nerve IV and depresses the medially rotated eye. It also rotates medially and abducts the eyeball.[9] (pp. 715–717)

Superior ophthalmic vein. This vein anastomoses with the facial vein and allows blood to flow in either direction because it has no valves. It crosses superior to the optic nerve through the superior orbital fissure ending in the cavernous sinus.[9] (p. 719)

Superior parietal lobule. This lobule is part of the parietal lobe. It is located in the posterior superior part of the parietal lobe immediately anterior to the parieto-occipital fissure. It is involved in sensory appreciation, such as stereognosis (recognition of objects by touch), graphesthesia (recognition of shapes written on the skin), and two-point discrimination.[3] (p. 404), [12] (pp. 17–18), [14] (p. 886)

Superior petrosal sinus. This sinus lies in the petrous portion of the temporal bone. Along with the inferior petrosal sinus, it drains the cavernous sinus and connects it with the sigmoid and transverse sinuses.[25] (p. 252)

Superior rectus muscle. This is one of the four rectus muscles: superior, inferior, medial, and lateral. All of these muscles arise from a common tendinous ring that surrounds the optic canal. It is innervated by the oculomotor nerve (cranial nerve III) and serves to elevate, adduct, and medially rotate the eye.[9] (pp. 715–717)

Superior sagittal sinus. This sinus drains blood from the brain by way of cerebral veins. It drains CSF from the subarachnoid space through the arachnoid villi, which project into the dural venous sinuses.[11] (pp. 292, 439)

Superior temporal gyrus. This gyrus is part of the temporal lobe on the lateral surface of the brain, and the most superior of three gyri that run parallel to the sylvian fissure. On the superior surface are a series of obliquely oriented gyri termed "the transverse temporal gyri of Heschl" that form the primary auditory cortex. The lateral surface of this gyrus in the dominant hemisphere is part of Wernicke's area, which is involved in receptive language functions.[1] (p. 161)

Superior temporal sulcus. This sulcus is located on the temporal lobe on the lateral surface of the brain and serves to separate the superior and middle temporal gyri.[1] (p. 161)

Supramarginal gyrus. This gyrus makes up

the anterior part of the inferior parietal lobule. It is believed to be involved in somatosensory and visual integration. In the dominant hemisphere it plays a role in the comprehension of written language.[3 (p. 409), 6 (pp. 18–20), 7 (pp. 405–407)]

Suprasellar (chiasmatic) cistern. This cistern is a large subarachnoid space located above the pituitary fossa and containing the optic nerves, chiasm, and proximal optic tracts, as well as the circle of Willis and the pituitary stalk.[3 (p. 438)]

Sylvian fissure (lateral sulcus or fissure). This fissure is a CSF-filled subarachnoid space that separates the temporal lobe from the frontal and parietal lobes.[19 (pp. 257–258)]

Teeth. The teeth form the superior and inferior dental arches composed of an outer portion, the crown, and a root imbedded in bone. These represent the organs of mastication and are influential in the articulation of speech.[8 (pp. 460–461)]

Tegmentum. The tegmentum refers to the dorsal parts of the pons and midbrain contributing structurally to the floor of the fourth ventricle. It includes the red nuclei, the substantia nigra, the periaqueductal gray, and fiber tracts.[12 (pp. 88, 108)]

Temporal bone. This is an irregular bone that forms part of the lateral surface and base of the skull. It contains the organs of hearing.[14 (p. 219)]

Temporal horn of lateral ventricle. This part of the ventricular system is an anteroinferior extension from the trigone of the lateral ventricle into the temporal lobe. Anteriorly, the shape is changed by the hippocampus, which protrudes into the lumen from the ventricular floor and results in a crescentic slit. The medial superior border is called the supracornual or medial cleft and it contains the choroid plexus located between the hippocampus and the tail of the caudate nucleus.[10 (pp. 76–77)]

Temporal lobe. The temporal lobe contains the primary auditory cortex, auditory and visual association areas, and several elements of the limbic system, including the amygdala, the parahippocampal gyrus, and the hippocampus. These limbic system structures mediate emotions, visceral responses, learning, and memory.[6 (pp. 21–22)]

Temporalis muscle. This muscle is one of the four pairs of the muscles of mastication, the other three being masseter, medial pterygoid, and lateral pterygoid. It assists in jaw closure and is innervated by the mandibular division of the trigeminal nerve.[8 (pp. 255–268)]

Tentorium cerebelli. This is a tent-shaped dural reflection that separates the occipital lobes from the cerebellum. It defines the intracranial supratentorial and infratentorial compartments and contains the dural sinuses that provide venous drainage for the brain.[14 (p. 219)]

Thalamus. The hypothalamus and the thalamus form the diencephalon. The thalamus is a collection of more than 20 smaller nuclei that serve as the main relay centers between the cortex and lower structures, including the basal ganglia, the cerebellum, the brainstem, and the spinal cord. There are three classes of thalamic nuclei: specific sensory relay nuclei; motor nuclei; and nonspecific association nuclei. All sensory systems (with the exception of olfaction) relay information to specialized cortical areas by way of the specific sensory relay nuclei of the thalamus. The motor nuclei interconnect the frontal cortices with the cerebellum and basal ganglia. Association nuclei interconnect cortical association regions and the limbic system with association cortices. In addition, there is a group of intrinsic nuclei without cortical connections and a series of nuclei that are part of the ascending reticular activating system. Connections between the thalamus and cortical areas are reciprocal, with feedback pathways appearing to provide the cerebral cortex with a mechanism for control of its inputs.[6 (p. 234), 20 (pp. 258–263)]

Third ventricle. The third ventricle transmits CSF from the lateral ventricles through the foramen of Monro to the fourth ventricle through the cerebral aqueduct. It is closed at the top by a thin, narrow velum interpositum and is bounded laterally by the thalami, which join medially at the massa intermedia and bridge the middle of this ventricle.[5] (p. 103)

Transverse venous sinus.   This sinus is one of the dural sinuses and it lies between the inner and outer layers of the dura. It contains no valves and provides venous drainage for the brain. The transverse sinus drains the confluence of sinuses (torcular Herophili). It extends anteriorly and laterally around the skull base through the inferior margin of the petrous bone, and enlarges inferiorly to form the sigmoid sinus.[1] (pp. 187–188), [25] (p. 251)

Trigeminal nerve (cranial nerve V).   This is the largest cranial nerve. It provides sensation to the face, most of the scalp, and the teeth, as well as the nasal and oral cavities. It divides into three branches: ophthalmic, maxillary, and mandibular nerves. It also provides motor innervation to the muscles of mastication.[1] (p. 404), [4] (p. 1059)

Trigeminal nucleus.   This is one of four cranial nerve nuclei within the general visceral brainstem nuclear column comprised of: the trigeminal motor nucleus, the facial motor nucleus, the nucleus ambiguus, and the accessory nucleus. It contains motor neurons with fibers in the trigeminal (V) nerve with principal innervation to the muscles of mastication.[2] (pp. 322–333)

Trigone of the lateral ventricle.   The trigone is that portion of the lateral ventricle (ependymal-lined cavity of each hemisphere filled with CSF) where the body, temporal, and occipital horns join to form a common cavity.[10] (pp. 74–75), [11] (p. 283), [12] (pp. 253–256)

Trochlear nerve (cranial nerve IV).   The trochlear is the smallest of the cranial nerves. It innervates the superior oblique muscle for movement of the eye down and out (abduction).[1] (p. 410)

Trochlear nucleus.   This nucleus is the second member of the general somatic motor column (oculomotor nucleus, trochlear nucleus, abducens nucleus, and hypoglossal nucleus) containing the motor neurons projecting peripherally through the trochlear nerve. The trochlear nerve is the only cranial nerve exiting from the dorsal brainstem. It allows for movement of the eye down and out (abduction).[1] (p. 41), [2] (pp. 322–333)

Tuber cinereum.   The tuber cinereum is the region bounded by the mamillary bodies, optic chiasm, and the origin of the optic tracts. It surrounds the pituitary stalk and is characterized by a swelling. Underneath this swelling are most of the hypothalamic nuclei that regulate the release of the anterior pituitary hormones.[2] (p. 350), [12] (p. 196)

Uncus of temporal lobe.   The uncus is the anterior part of the parahippocampal gyrus of the temporal lobe, forming a medial convex prominence. It is used as an anatomic landmark and contains cortical areas involved in olfactory and limbic functions.[2] (pp. 200–202), [6] (pp. 21–22)

Vagus nerve (cranial nerve X).   The vagus has the most extensive course and distribution of any cranial nerve passing down the neck within the carotid sheath to the thorax, and then to the abdomen. It is attached to the medulla oblongata by 8 to 10 rootlets with fibers connected to four nuclei in the medulla oblongata: dorsal nucleus, nucleus ambiguus, nucleus of the tractus solitarius, and spinal nucleus of the trigeminal nerve. It provides (1) general visceral efferent innervation to the thorax and most of the abdomen; (2) special visceral efferent innervation to the pharynx and larynx; and (3) general visceral afferent fibers which carry sensory information from the pharynx, larynx, thorax, and abdomen. It has a general somatic afferent component that innervates the external ear and a special visceral afferent component that innervates taste buds on the epiglottis (primarily of importance in infancy).[1] (p. 423), [4] (pp. 1076–1080)

Ventral lateral nucleus.   The ventral anterior nucleus of the thalamus and the ventral lateral nucleus form the motor functional division of the thalamic nuclei. The ventral lateral nucleus conveys motor information from the cerebellum and globus pallidus to the precentral motor cortex.[3] (pp. 144–145), [22] (pp. 90–92)

Ventral posterolateral nucleus.   This thalamic nucleus is the sensory relay nucleus for the somatosensory system. It gives rise to somatotopic projections to the primary somatosensory cortex of the postcentral gyrus. It is noteworthy that the perceptual mechanisms of pain are believed to be associated with thalamic processes rather than activity of the primary somatosensory cortex.[3] (pp. 144–145), [22] (pp. 90–92)

Ventral spinothalamic tract. This fiber pathway transmits light touch information to the thalamus from the contralateral side of the body. Its cells of origin are located in the posterior gray horns of the spinal cord (lamina VI and VII). These fibers decussate at the level of the spinal cord in the anterior white commissure.[2] (p. 125), [3] (p. 193), [20] (pp. 180–181)

Ventral trigeminothalamic tract. The ventral trigeminothalamic tract is similar to the anterolateral spinothalamic tract and courses through the midbrain to the thalamus, transmitting contralateral pain and temperature from the face.[2] (p. 307), [3] (p. 193)

Vertebral artery. This artery originates as the first large branch of either subclavian artery. It generally ascends through the foramina in the transverse process of the cervical vertebrae with the exception of the seventh. It then courses behind the lateral mass of the atlas and enters the skull through the foramen magnum, joining the opposite side at the lower border of the pons to form the basilar artery. The vertebral artery gives branches to the head and neck, including spinal and muscular arteries. The cranial branches of the vertebral artery include meningeal, posterior spinal, anterior spinal, medullary, and the posterior inferior cerebellar arteries.[4] (pp. 694–696), [10] (pp. 228–229)

Vestibule. This is an oval bony chamber containing the utricle and saccule. It is continuous anteriorly with the bony cochlea, posteriorly with the semicircular canals, and it communicates with the posterior fossa by means of the vestibular aqueduct. It is important in maintaining balance and equilibrium.[9] (pp. 775–776)

Vitreous body (eye). This body is made up of material that fills the eyeball posterior to the lens. It consists of a jellylike material referred to as the vitreous humor. This colorless and transparent gel is located within the vitreous chamber, which is the space between the lens and the retina. This "body" forms most of the eyeball, transmits light, holds the retina in place, and provides support for the lens.[9] (p 714)

Vomer. The vomer is a bony structure forming the back and lower part of the nasal septum.[8] (p. 123)

Wernicke's area. The broad definition of Wernicke's area includes the angular and part of the supramarginal gyri that constitutes Brodmann's area 39 and parts of 40. [A somewhat restricted definition that is used for Wernicke's area includes only part of the superior and middle temporal gyri (part of Brodmann's areas 21 and 22)]. Wernicke's area is located in the dominant hemisphere and is involved in understanding of spoken or written language as well as gestures and musical sounds.[1] (p. 169)

Zygomatic process of frontal bone. This process is located inferiorly on the frontal bone. It forms the lateral aspect of the superior orbit articulating with the zygomatic bone.[4] (p. 333)

Sagittal Views

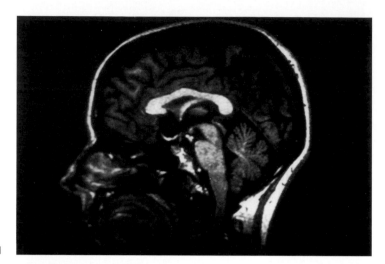

MRI

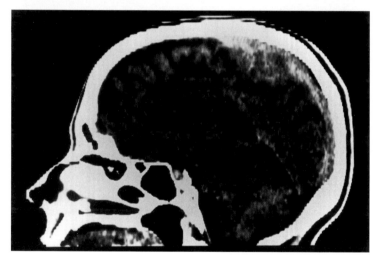

CT

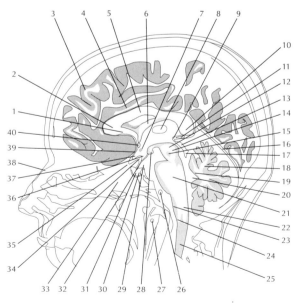

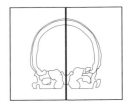

Sagittal 1

1. *Rostrum of corpus callosum.* Forms the anterior wall of the third ventricle.[12 (pp. 246, 248)]

2. *Genu of corpus callosum.* Connects the frontal lobes.[2 (pp. 51, 31), 12 (p. 248), 15 (p. 365), 19 (p. 269)]

3. *Superior frontal gyrus.* Participates in the control and initiation of voluntary movements and is involved in personality, insight, and judgment.[6 (pp. 18–20), 18 (p. 674), 19 (p. 260)]

4. *Cingulate gyrus.* Plays a role in emotional behavior, the autonomic nervous system, learning and memory.[12 (p. 272), 18 (pp. 255, 674)]

5. *Body of the corpus callosum.* Interconnects the cerebral hemispheres.[2 (pp. 51, 131), 12 (p. 248), 16 (p. 33)]

6. *Fornix.* Efferent tract of the hippocampus projecting to the mamillary bodies.[11 (p. 276), 12 (pp. 268–269), 19 (p. 269)]

7. *Paraventricular nucleus.* Has neurosecretory functions and produces the neurohormones vasopressin and oxytocin.[1 (pp. 384–385), 2 (p. 354)]

8. *Thalamus.* Serves as the main relay center for the nervous system.[6 (p. 234), 20 (pp. 258–263)]

9. *Posterior commissure.* Contains collections of nerve cells, which include papillary light reflex involvement.[11 (p. 246), 12 (p. 195)]

10. *Splenium of corpus callosum.* Enlargement of the corpus callosum posteriorly connecting the occipital lobes.[11 (pp. 244–245), 12 (p. 248), 19 (p. 269)]

11. *Pineal gland.* Associated with the mechanisms that regulate circadian rhythm.[1 (p. 149), 8 (435–438)]

12. *Midbrain (mesencephalon).* Involved in the control of eye movements, motor control, and contains relay nuclei.[5 (p. 276)]

13. *Superior colliculus.* Receives visual signals directly from the retina or indirectly from the visual cortex, and is essential for rapid eye movements.[1 (pp. 245–246, 412)]

14. *Tegmentum.* Dorsal part of the pons and midbrain contributing structurally to the floor of the fourth ventricle.[12 (pp. 88, 108)]

15. *Red nucleus.* Relays impulses from the cerebral and cerebellar cortex to the spinal cord.[1 (p. 353), 19 (pp. 435–436), 20 (pp. 225–226, 250)]

16. *Straight venous sinus.* Provides cerebral venous drainage.[7 (p. 61), 15 (p. 440–441)]

17. *Inferior colliculus.* Participates in auditory pathways and relays impulses to the medial geniculate body.[2 (p. 178), 12 (p. 90), 20 (p. 372)]

18. *Cerebellum.* Primarily involved in motor function through the maintenance of equilibrium and the coordination of muscle action.[1 (pp. 15, 132–133), 4 (pp. 338–340), 6 (pp. 18–20)]

19. *Superior medullary velum.* Forms part of the roof of the fourth ventricle.[1 (pp. 136–137)]

20. *Fourth ventricle.* Cavity filled with cerebrospinal fluid (CSF).[7 (p. 70), 13 (p. 97)]

21. *Pons.* Contains neural circuits that transmit information between the spinal cord and

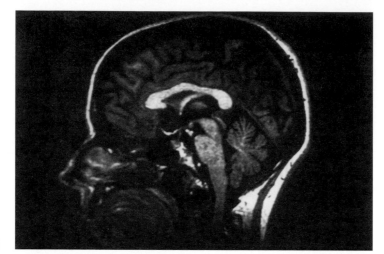

MRI

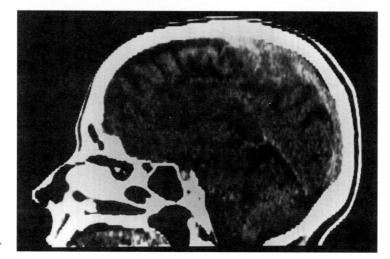

CT

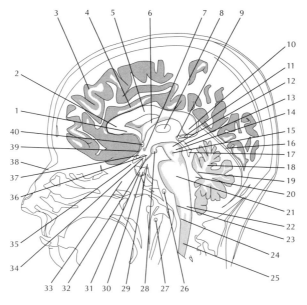

higher brain regions. Regulates level of arousal, blood pressure, and respiration.[2] [(p. 9),] [11] [(p. 181)]

22. *Medulla oblongata (myelencephalon or medulla).* Involved in digestion, breathing, blood pressure, and heart rate.[1] [(pp. 15, 132–133),] [2] [(p. 9),] [13] [(pp. 7, 61),] [15] [(p. 9)]

23. *Pyramid.* Contains the lateral and ventral corticospinal tracts as well as the corticobulbar tracts.[2] [(p. 229)]

24. *Pyramidal decussation.* Allows one side of the brain to control the opposite side of the body.[12] [(p. 336)]

25. *Spinal cord.* Innervates the motor and sensory areas of the body.[1] [(p. 117),] [4] [(p. 864)]

26. *Basilar artery.* Blood supply to upper medulla, pons, cerebellum, inner ear, occipital lobe, and part of the temporal lobe.[15] [(p. 1042)]

27. *Anterior arch of the atlas.* Joins the lateral masses of the first cervical vertebrae.[4] [(pp. 273–274),] [8] [(pp. 129–130)]

28. *Mamillary body.* Receives hippocampal input.[1] [(p. 386),] [2] [(367–368, 381, 392)]

29. *Suprasellar (chiasmatic) cistern.* Subarachnoid space located above the pituitary fossa.[3] [(p. 438)]

30. *Neurohypophysis (posterior lobe of the pituitary gland).* A neurohemal organ consisting of neurosecretory axons ending on capillary blood vessels.[12] [(pp. 196, 201–203)]

31. *Anterior lobe of the pituitary.* Produces numerous hormones.[2] [(p. 350),] [3] [(pp. 421–424),] [12] [(pp. 201–203)]

32. *Infundibulum (pituitary stalk, hypophyseal stalk).* Connects the pituitary gland to the hypothalamus.[2] [(p. 355),] [12] [(p. 196),] [15] [(p. 739)]

33. *Sphenoid sinus.* Acts as a resonator to the voice.[23] [(pp. 734–736)]

34. *Optic chiasm.* Convergence of the optic nerves.[2] [(p. 143),] [11] [(p. 227)]

35. *Chiasmatic cistern.* Ventral CSF-filled subarachnoid space.[10] [(pp. 113–120)]

36. *Infundibular recess.* CSF-filled recess in the floor of the third ventricle.[2] [(p. 350)]

37. *Optic recess.* Anterior projection of the third ventricle.[3] [(p. 315)]

38. *Nasal bone.* Forms the bridge of the nose.[9] [(p. 651)]

39. *Lamina terminalis.* Provides input to the hypothalamus regarding blood volume and blood pressure control.[2] [(pp. 36, 356),] [12] [(pp. 196–197)]

40. *Anterior commissure.* A neocortical "corpus callosum."[2] [(pp. 249–250),] [11] [(p. 246)]

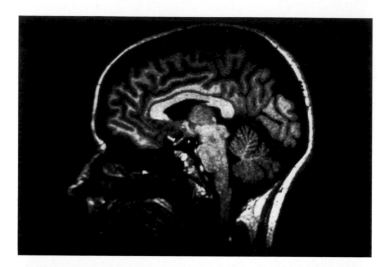

MRI

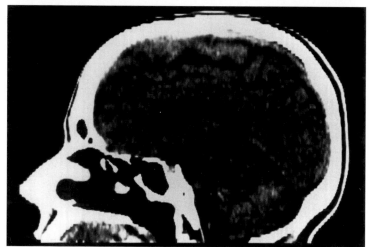

CT

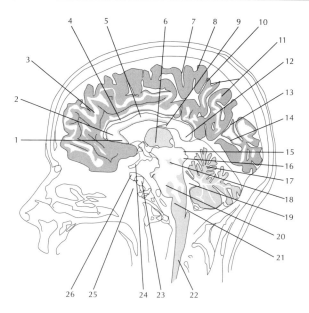

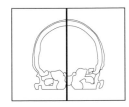

Sagittal 2

1. *Rostrum of corpus callosum.* Forms the anterior wall of the third ventricle.[12] (pp. 246, 248)

2. *Genu of corpus callosum.* Connects the frontal lobes.[2] (p. 51), [12] (p. 248), [15] (p. 365), [19] (p. 269)

3. *Superior frontal gyrus.* Participates in the control and initiation of voluntary movements and is involved in personality, insight, and judgment.[6] (pp. 18–20), [18] (p. 674), [19] (p. 260)

4. *Callosal sulcus.* Separates the cingulate gyrus from the corpus callosum.[11] (p. 236)

5. *Body of the corpus callosum.* Interconnects the cerebral hemispheres.[2] (pp. 51, 131), [12] (p. 51), [16] (p. 33)

6. *Thalamus.* Serves as the main relay center for the nervous system.[6] (p. 234), [20] (pp. 258–263)

7. *Central sulcus.* Separates the primary motor cortex (frontal) from the primary somatosensory cortex (parietal).[19] (p. 257)

8. *Paracentral lobule.* Medial extension of the precentral (motor) and postcentral (sensory) gyri.[6] (pp. 18–20)

9. *Posterior commissure.* Contains collections of nerve cells, which include pupillary light reflex involvement.[2] (p. 195), [11] (p. 246)

10. *Parietal occipital sulcus.* Separates the parietal and occipital lobes.[11] (p.233), [19] (p.259)

11. *Precuneus (quadrate lobe).* Involved in complex sensory appreciation, language comprehension, and may be involved in complex aspects of orientation to time and space.[3] (p. 404), [6] (pp. 18–20), [14] (p. 1249)

12. *Splenium of corpus callosum.* Enlargement of corpus callosum posteriorly connecting the occipital lobe.[11] (pp. 244–245), [12] (p. 248), [19] (p. 269)

13. *Parietal occipital sulcus.* Separates the parietal and occipital lobes.[11] (p. 233), [19] (p. 259)

14. *Calcarine sulcus.* Marks the visual cortex.[11] (pp. 242, 260), [12] (pp. 217–218)

15. *Superior colliculus.* Receives visual signals directly from the retina or indirectly from the visual cortex and is essential for rapid eye movements.[1] (pp. 245–246, 412)

16. *Inferior colliculus.* Participates in auditory pathways, and relays impulses to the medial geniculate body.[2] (p. 178), [12] (p. 90), [20] (p. 372)

17. *Cerebellum.* Primarily involved in motor function through the maintenance of equilibrium and the coordination of muscle action.[1] (pp. 15, 132–133), [4] (pp. 338–340), [6] (pp. 18–20)

18. *Red nucleus.* Relays impulses from the cerebral and cerebellar cortex to the spinal cord.[1] (p. 353), [2] (pp. 225–226, 250), [16] (pp. 435–436)

19. *Fourth ventricle.* Cavity filled with cerebrospinal fluid.[7] (p. 70), [13] (p. 97)

20. *Pons.* Contains neural circuits that transmit information between the spinal cord and higher brain regions. Regulates levels of arousal, blood pressure, and respiration.[2] (p. 90), [11] (p. 181)

21. *Medulla oblongata (myelencephalon of medulla).* Involved in digestion, breathing, blood pressure, and heart rate.[1] (pp. 15, 132–133), [2] (p. 9), [13] (pp. 7, 61), [15] (p. 9)

37

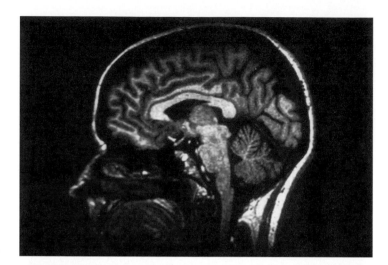

MRI

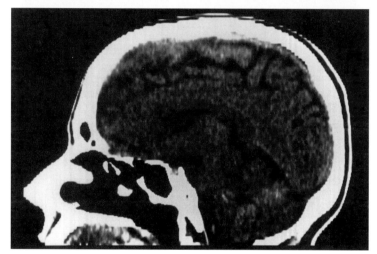

CT

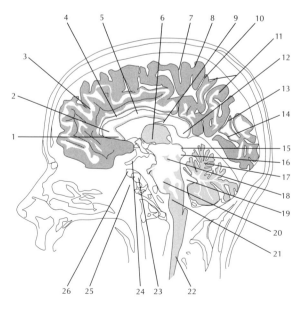

22. *Spinal cord.* Innervates the motor and sensory areas of the body.[1] (p. 117), [4] (p. 864)

23. *Neurohypophysis (posterior lobe of the pituitary gland).* A neurohemal organ consisting of neurosecretory axons ending on capillary blood vessels.[12] (pp. 196, 201–203)

24. *Optic nerve (cranial nerve II).* Nerve of sight.[7] (pp. 221, 227)

25. *Sphenoid sinus.* Acts as a resonator to the voice.[23] (pp. 734–736)

26. *Anterior lobe of pituitary.* Produces numerous hormones.[2] (p. 350), [3] (pp. 421, 422), [12] (pp. 201, 203)

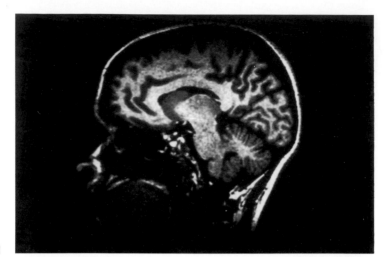

MRI

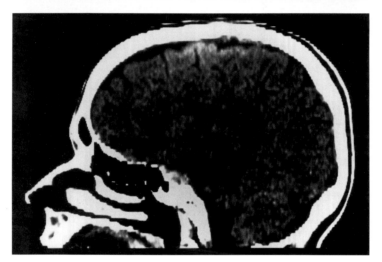

CT

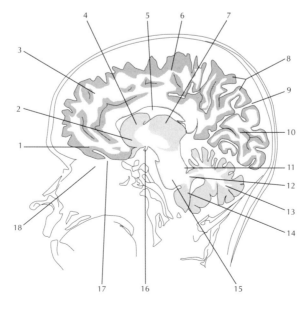

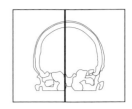

Sagittal 3

1. *Orbital gyrus.* Involved in the conscious perception of odors.[1 (pp. 160, 296, 493)]

2. *Lentiform nucleus.* Receiving station for the basal ganglia.[1 (p. 336), 12 (p. 207)]

3. *Frontal lobe.* Involved in personality, insight, and foresight; initiation of voluntary movements; written and spoken language.[6 (pp. 18–20)]

4. *Caudate nucleus.* Involved in cognitive functions and movement.[6 (p. 304), 7 (pp. 11), 12 (pp. 207–212), 15 (pp. 306–307), 18 (pp. 523–524)]

5. *Lateral ventricle.* Ependymal-lined C-shaped cavity of each hemisphere filled with cerebrospinal fluid.[11 (p. 183), 12 (pp. 253–256)]

6. *Parietal lobe.* The postcentral gyrus is the first somesthetic area; however, it also has a motor component. The association cortex allows for processing the significance of sensory data, including prior experience.[9 (p. 693), 12 (pp. 232–235)]

7. *Thalamus.* Serves as the main relay center for the nervous system.[6 (p. 234), 20 (pp. 258–363)]

8. *Precuneus.* Involved in complex sensory appreciation, language comprehension, and may be involved in complex aspects of orientation to time and space.[6 (pp. 18–20), 13 (p. 404), 14 (p. 1249)]

9. *Parietal occipital sulcus.* Separates the parietal and occipital lobes.[11 (p. 233), 19 (p. 259)]

10. *Occipital lobe.* Involved in the higher order processing of visual information.[6 (pp. 21–22)]

11. *Superior cerebellar peduncle.* Connects the cerebellum to the midbrain.[2 (pp. 242, 249), 11 (p. 13), 12 (pp. 104–105), 20 (p. 326)]

12. *Middle cerebellar peduncle.* Connects cerebellum to pons, relaying input from the contralateral cerebral cortex to the lateral lobe of the cerebellum.[2 (pp. 242, 249), 11 (p. 13), 12 (pp. 104–105)]

13. *Cerebellum.* Primarily involved in motor function through the maintenance of equilibrium and the coordination of muscle action.[1 (pp. 15, 132–133), 4 (pp. 338–340), 6 (pp. 18–20)]

14. *Inferior cerebellar peduncle.* Connects the cerebellum to the medulla, and is important in maintaining equilibrium.[2 (pp. 242, 249), 11 (p. 13), 12 (pp. 104–105), 20 (pp. 326–327)]

15. *Pons.* Contains neural circuits that transmit information between the spinal cord and higher brain regions. Regulates levels of arousal, blood pressure, and respiration.[2 (p. 9), 11 (p. 181)]

16. *Optic tract.* Transmission of visual impulses from the retina.[15 (p. 424), 19 (p. 399)]

17. *Cribriform plate.* Forms the roof of the nasal fossa.[4 (p. 334–336), 8 (p. 119)]

18. *Ethmoid bone.* Forms the roof of the nasal fossa.[4 (pp. 334–336), 8 (p. 119)]

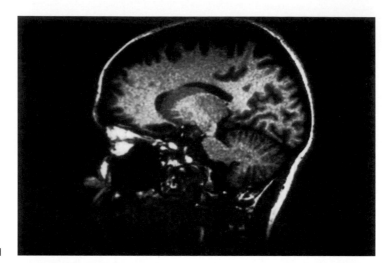

MRI

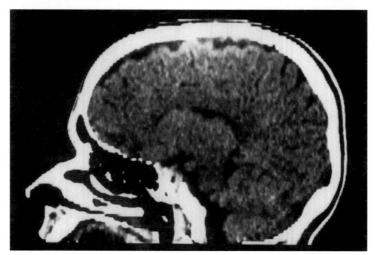

CT

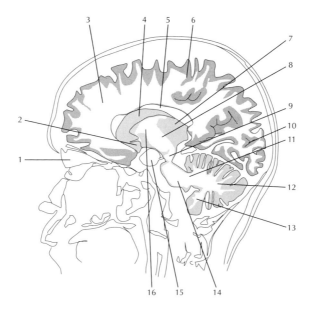

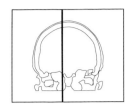

Sagittal 4

1. *Orbital fat.* Provides cushioning and support of the eye.[25] (p. 188)

2. *Putamen.* Involved in motor function.[6] (p. 304), [7] (p. 11)

3. *Frontal lobe.* Involved in personality, insight, and foresight; initiation of voluntary movements; written and spoken language.[6] (pp. 18–20)

4. *Caudate nucleus.* Involved in cognitive functions and movement.[6] (p. 304), [7] (p. 11), [12] (pp. 207–212), [15] (pp. 306–307), [18] (pp. 523–525)

5. *Lateral ventricle.* Ependymal-lined C-shaped cavity of each hemisphere filled with cerebrospinal fluid.[11] (p. 183), [12] (pp. 253–256)

6. *Parietal lobe.* The postcentral gyrus is the first somesthetic area; however, it also has a motor component. The association cortex allows for processing the significance of sensory data, including prior experience.[9] (p. 693), [12] (pp. 232–235)

7. *Thalamus.* Serves as the main relay center for the nervous system.[6] (p. 234), [20] (pp. 258–263)

8. *Internal capsule—-posterior limb.* Contains fibers of general sensation.[7] (p. 12), [11] (p. 249), [16] (p. 538)

9. *Cerebral peduncle.* Forms both sides of the midbrain, excluding the tectum.[2] (p. 226), [12] (p. 108)

10. *Occipital lobe.* Involved in the higher order processing of visual information.[6] (pp. 21–22)

11. *Middle cerebellar peduncle.* Connects cerebellum to pons, relaying input from the contralateral cerebral cortex to the lateral lobe of the cerebellum.[2] (pp. 242, 249), [11] (p. 13), [12] (pp. 104–105)

12. *Cerebellum.* Primarily involved in motor function through the maintenance of equilibrium and the coordination of muscle action.[2] (pp. 242, 249), [11] (p. 13), [12] (p. 104–105), [20] (pp. 326–327)

13. *Inferior cerebellar peduncle.* Connects the cerebellum to the medulla and is important in maintaining equilibrium.[2] (pp. 242, 249), [11] (p. 13), [12] (pp. 104–105), [20] (pp. 326–327)

14. *Pons.* Contains neural circuits that transmit information between the spinal cord and higher brain regions. Regulates levels of arousal, blood pressure, and respiration.[2] (p. 9), [11] (p. 181)

15. *Uncus of temporal lobe.* Anterior part of the parahippocampal gyrus, used as an anatomic landmark.[2] (pp. 200–202), [6] (pp. 21–22)

16. *Internal capsule—genu.* Contains corticobulbar and corticoreticular connection fibers.[7] (p. 12), [11] (p. 249), [16] (p. 538)

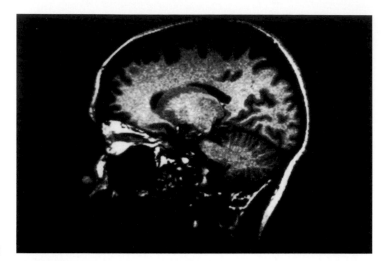

MRI

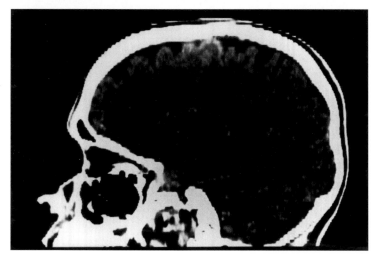

CT

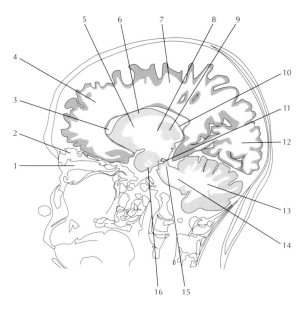

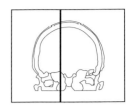

Sagittal 5

1. *Medial rectus muscle.* Rotates the eye so that the cornea is directed medially.[9] (p. 715), [25] (p. 189)

2. *Orbital fat.* Provides cushioning and support of the eye.[25] (p. 188)

3. *Lateral ventricle.* Ependymal-lined C-shaped cavity of each hemisphere filled with cerebrospinal fluid.[11] (p. 183), [12] (pp. 253–256)

4. *Frontal lobe.* Involved in personality, insight, and foresight; initiation of voluntary movements; written and spoken language.[6] (pp. 18–20)

5. *Internal capsule—anterior limb.* Connects subcortical nuclei with the cerebral cortex and the cerebral cortex with subcortical structures.[7] (p. 12), [11] (p. 249), [16] (p. 538)

6. *Caudate nucleus.* Involved in cognitive functions and movement.[6] (p. 304), [7] (p. 11), [12] (pp. 207–212), [15] (pp. 306–307), [18] (pp. 523–524)

7. *Parietal lobe.* The postcentral gyrus is the first somesthetic area; however, it also has a motor component. The association cortex allows for processing the significance of sensory data, including prior experience.[9] (p. 693), [12] (pp. 232–235)

8. *Internal capsule—posterior limb.* Contains fibers of general sensation.[7] (p. 12), [11] (p. 249), [16] (p. 538)

9. *Thalamus.* Along with the posterolateral and dorsolateral nuclei, the thalamus forms the multimodal functional division of the thalamic nuclei.[3] (pp. 144–145), [22] (pp. 90–92)

10. *Stria terminalis.* Involved in the circuitry of the limbic system.[1] (p. 493)

11. *Medial lemniscus.* Transmits touch and proprioception for the contralateral side of the body.[1] (pp. 203–206)

12. *Occipital lobe.* Involved in the higher order processing of visual information.[6] (pp. 21–22)

13. *Cerebellum.* Primarily involved in motor function through the maintenance of equilibrium and the coordination of muscle action.[1] (pp. 24, 132–133), [4] (pp. 338–340), [6] (pp. 18–20)

14. *Middle cerebellar peduncle.* Connects cerebellum to pons, relaying input from the contralateral cerebral cortex to the lateral lobe of the cerebellum.[2] (pp. 242, 249), [11] (p. 13), [12] (pp. 104–105)

15. *Cerebral peduncle.* Forms both sides of the midbrain, excluding the tectum.[2] (p. 226), [12] (p. 108)

16. *Amygdala (amygdaloid complex).* Involved in olfactory perception, visceral function, and emotions.[2] (pp. 200–202)

MRI

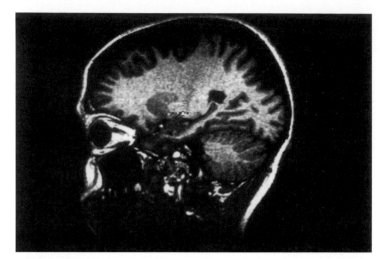

CT

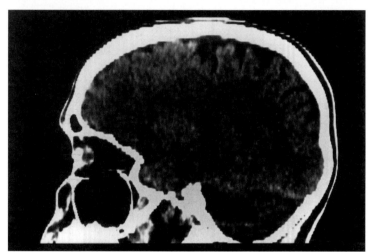

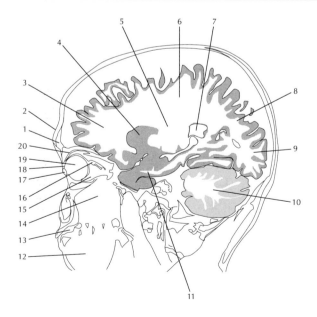

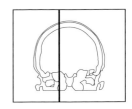

Sagittal 6

1. *Frontal sinus.* Acts as a resonator for the voice.[9] (pp. 760–762), [14] (p. 1424), [23] (pp. 734–736)

2. *Frontal bone.* Provides enclosure and protection of the brain.[24] (p. 170)

3. *Frontal lobe.* Involved in personality, insight, and foresight; initiation of voluntary movements; written and spoken language.[6] (pp. 18–20)

4. *Putamen.* Involved in motor function.[6] (p. 304), [7] (p. 11)

5. *Corona radiata.* Establishes reciprocal connections between the cerebral cortex and the thalamus.[12] (p. 351), [14] (p. 361)

6. *Parietal lobe.* The postcentral gyrus is the first somesthetic area; however, it also has a motor component. The association cortex allows for processing the significance of sensory data, including prior experience.[9] (p. 693), [12] (pp. 232–235)

7. *Trigone of the lateral ventricle.* Where the body and temporal and occipital horns join to form a common cavity.[10] (pp. 74–75), [11] (p. 283), [12] (pp. 253–256)

8. *Inferior parietal lobule.* May involve written, visual, and auditory language integration.[3] (p. 409), [6] (p. 20), [14] (p. 848)

9. *Occipital lobe.* Involved in the higher order processing of visual information.[6] (pp. 21–22)

10. *Cerebellum.* Primarily involved in motor function through the maintenance of equilibrium and the coordination of muscle action.[1] (pp. 15, 132–133), [4] (pp. 338–340), [6] (pp. 18–20)

11. *Temporal lobe.* Involved in emotions, visceral responses, learning, and memory.[6] (pp. 21–22)

12. *Body of the mandible.* Forms part of the lower jaw and face.[8] (pp. 121–123), [17] (p. 815)

13. *Maxilla.* Forms the upper jaw, most of the roof of the mouth, the floor and the lateral walls or the nasal cavity, and the floor of the orbit.[4] (pp. 338–340)

14. *Maxillary sinus.* Acts as a resonator to the voice.[23] (pp. 734–736)

15. *Inferior rectus muscle.* Serves to depress, adduct, and laterally rotate the eye.[9] (pp. 715–717)

16. *Optic nerve.* Nerve of sight.[7] (pp. 221, 227)

17. *Cornea.* Responsible for refraction of the light that enters the eye.[9] (p. 714)

18. *Globe.* Complex structure for vision.[8] (pp. 380–384), [25] (p. 188)

19. *Vitreous body (eye).* Forms most of the eyeball, transmits light, holds the retina in place, and provides support for the lens.[9] (p. 714)

20. *Superior rectus muscle.* Serves to elevate, adduct, and medially rotate the eye.[9] (pp. 715–717)

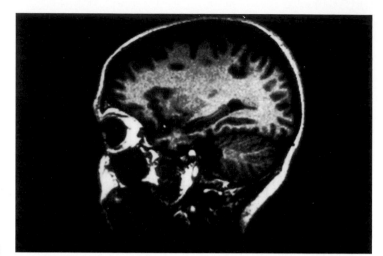

MRI

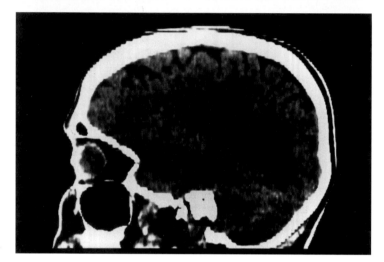

CT

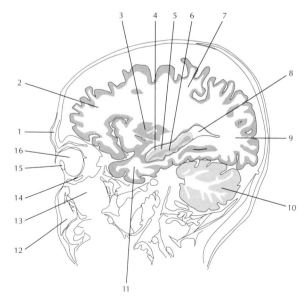

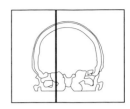

Sagittal 7

1. *Frontal bone.* Provides enclosure and protection of the brain.[24] (p. 170)

2. *Frontal lobe.* Involved in personality, insight, and foresight; initiation of voluntary movements; written and spoken language.[6] (pp. 18–20)

3. *Putamen.* Involved in motor function.[6] (p. 304), [7] (p. 11)

4. *Temporal horn of the lateral ventricle.* Anteroinferior extension from the trigone of the lateral ventricle into the temporal lobe.[10] (pp. 76–77)

5. *Hippocampus.* Plays a role in emotional behavior, regulation of the autonomic nervous system, learning, and memory.[15] (p. 307), [16] (pp. 630–631), [18] (pp. 255–256)

6. *Dentate gyrus.* Involved in memory and the emotions related to survival.[2] (p. 379), [12] (pp. 266–267), [13] (pp. 353—354)

7. *Parietal lobe.* The postcentral gyrus is the first somesthetic area; however, it also has a motor component. The association cortex allows for processing the significance of sensory data, including prior experience.[9] (p. 693), [12] (pp. 232–235)

8. *Trigone of the lateral ventricle.* Where the body and temporal and occipital horns join to form a common cavity.[10] (pp. 74–75), [11] (p. 283), [12] (pp. 253–256)

9. *Occipital lobe.* Involved in the higher order processing of visual information.[6] (pp. 21–22)

10. *Cerebellum.* Primarily involved in motor function through the maintenance of equilibrium and the coordination of muscle action.[1] (pp. 15, 132–133), [4] (pp. 338–340), [6] (pp. 18–20)

11. *Temporal lobe.* Involved in emotions, visceral responses, learning, and memory.[6] (pp. 21–22)

12. *Maxilla.* Forms the upper jaw, most of the roof of the mouth, the floor and the lateral walls of the nasal cavity, and the floor of the orbit.[4] (pp. 338–340)

13. *Maxillary sinus.* Acts as a resonator to the voice.[23] (pp. 734–736)

14. *Inferior oblique muscle.* Serves to elevate the medially rotated eye and to abduct and rotate the eye laterally.[9] (pp. 715–717)

15. *Lens.* Completes the refraction of entering light.[24] (pp. 283–287)

16. *Vitreous body (eye).* Forms most of the eyeball, transmits light, holds the retina in place, and provides support for the lens.[9] (p. 714)

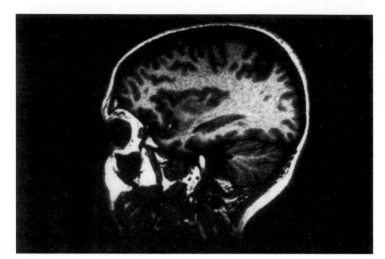

MRI

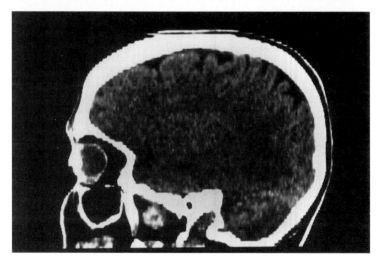

CT

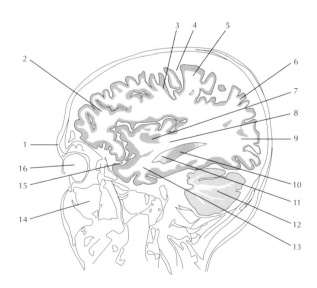

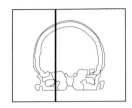

Sagittal 8

1. *Frontal bone.* Provides enclosure and protection of the brain.[24] (p. 170)

2. *Middle frontal gyrus.* Participates in the control and initiation of voluntary movements; involved in personality, insight, and foresight.[6] (p. 18)

3. *Precentral gyrus.* Location of the primary motor cortex.[1] (pp. 157, 326–327)

4. *Central sulcus.* Separates the primary motor cortex (frontal) from the primary somatosensory cortex (parietal).[19] (p. 257)

5. *Postcentral gyrus.* The area of the cortex associated with general sensory information.[6] (pp. 18–20)

6. *Inferior parietal lobule.* May involve written, visual, and auditory language integration.[3] (p. 409), [6] (p. 20), [14] (p. 848)

7. *Putamen.* Involved in motor function.[6] (p. 304), [7] (p. 11)

8. *Optic radiation.* Maintains a precise visuotopic organization from the lateral geniculate body to the primary visual cortex.[1] (p. 240)

9. *Occipital lobe.* Involved in the higher order processing of visual information.[6] (pp. 21–22)

10. *Hippocampus.* Plays a role in emotional behavior, regulation of the autonomic nervous system, learning, and memory.[15] (p. 307), [16] (pp. 630–631), [18] (pp. 255–256)

11. *Temporal horn of lateral ventricle.* Anterior inferior extension from the trigone of the lateral ventricle into the temporal lobe.[21] (pp. 76–77)

12. *Cerebellar hemisphere.* Involved with movements of the extremities and fine coordinated movements.[3] (p. 283), [12] (p. 175), [15] (pp. 633–634)

13. *Temporal lobe.* Involved in emotions, visceral responses, learning, and memory.[6] (pp. 21–22)

14. *Maxillary sinus.* Acts as a resonator to the voice.[23] (pp. 734–736)

15. *Sylvian fissure (lateral sulcus or fissure).* Separates temporal lobe from frontal and parietal lobes.[19] (pp. 257–258)

16. *Vitreous body (eye).* Forms most of the eyeball, transmits light, holds the retina in place, and provides support for the lens.[9] (p. 714)

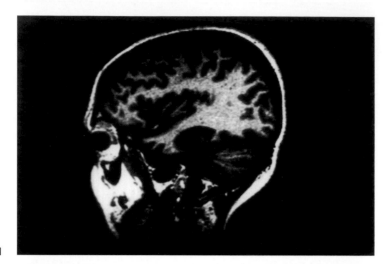

MRI

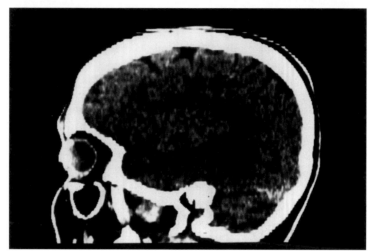

CT

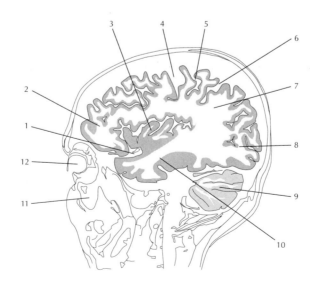

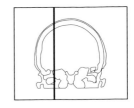

Sagittal 9

1. *Sylvian fissure.* Separates temporal lobe from frontal and parietal lobes.[19 (pp. 257–258)]
2. *Middle frontal gyrus.* Participates in the control and initiation of voluntary movements; involved in personality, insight, and foresight.[6 (p. 18)]
3. *Superior temporal gyrus.* The primary auditory cortex.[1 (p. 161)]
4. *Precentral sulcus.* Anterior to the precentral gyrus.[6 (pp. 18–20)]
5. *Central sulcus.* Separates the primary motor cortex (frontal) from the primary somatosensory cortex (parietal).[19 (p. 257)]
6. *Postcentral sulcus.* Lies behind the postcentral gyrus.[6 (pp. 18–20)]
7. *Parietal lobe.* The postcentral gyrus is the first somesthetic area; however, it also has a motor component. The association cortex allows for processing the significance of sensory data, including prior experience.[9 (p. 693), 12 (pp. 232–235)]
8. *Occipital lobe.* Involved in the higher order processing of visual information.[6 (pp. 21—22)]
9. *Cerebellar hemisphere.* Involved with movements of the extremities and fine coordinated movements.[3 (p. 383), 12 (p. 175), 15 (pp. 633–634)]
10. *Temporal lobe.* Involved in emotions, visceral responses, learning, and memory.[6 (pp. 21–22)]
11. *Maxillary sinus.* Acts as a resonator to the voice.[23 (pp. 734–736)]
12. *Vitreous body (eye).* Forms most of the eyeball, transmits light, holds the retina in place, and provides support for the lens.[9 (p. 714)]

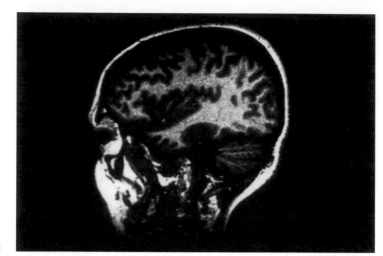

MRI

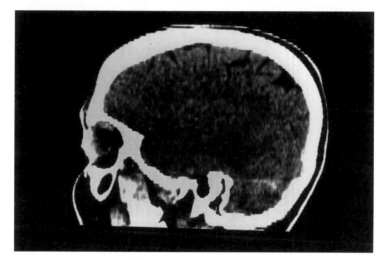

CT

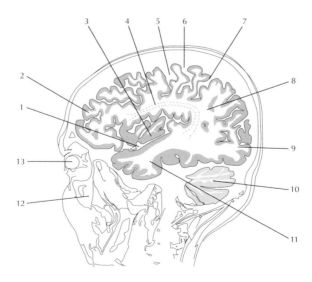

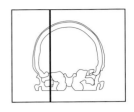

Sagittal 10

1. *Sylvian fissure (lateral sulcus or fissure).* Separates temporal lobe from frontal and parietal lobes.[19] [(pp. 257–258)]

2. *Middle frontal gyrus.* Participates in the control and initiation of voluntary movements; involved in personality, insight, and foresight.[6] [(p. 18)]

3. *Insular cortex (island of Reil).* Associated with visceral functions, and anteriorly contains the cortical gustatory (taste) area.[12] [(pp. 209–213), 19 (p. 294), 23 (p. 196)]

4. *Arcuate fasciculus.* Connects Wernicke's and Broca's areas.[2] [(p. 184)]

5. *Precentral sulcus.* Anterior to the precentral gyrus.[6] [(pp. 18–20)]

6. *Central sulcus.* Separates the primary motor cortex (frontal) from the primary somatosensory cortex (parietal).[19] [(p. 257)]

7. *Postcentral sulcus.* Lies behind the postcentral gyrus.[6] [(pp. 18–20)]

8. *Parietal lobe.* The postcentral gyrus is the first somesthetic area; however, it also has a motor component. The association cortex allows for processing the significance of sensory data including prior experience.[9] [(p. 693), 12 (pp. 232–235)]

9. *Occipital lobe.* Involved in the higher order processing of visual information.[6] [(pp. 21–22)]

10. *Cerebellar hemisphere.* Involved with the movements of the extremities and fine coordinated movements.[3] [(p. 283), 12 (p. 175), 15 (pp. 633–634)]

11. *Temporal lobe.* Involved in emotions, visceral responses, learning, and memory.[6] [(pp. 21—22)]

12. *Maxillary sinus.* Acts as a resonator to the voice.[23] [(pp. 734–736)]

13. *Vitreous body (eye).* Forms most of the eyeball, transmits light, holds the retina in place, and provides support for the lens.[9] [(p. 714)]

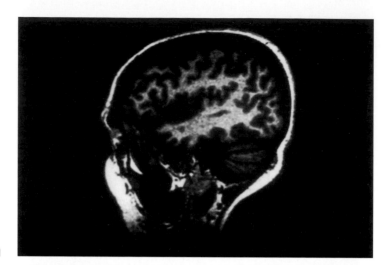

MRI

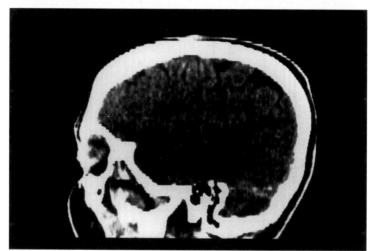

CT

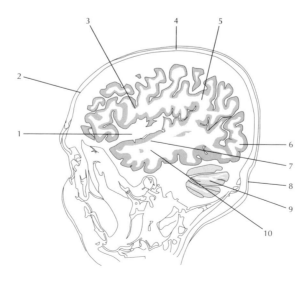

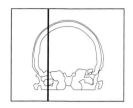

Sagittal 11

1. *Sylvian fissure (lateral sulcus or fissure).* Separates temporal lobe from frontal and parietal lobes.[19 (pp. 257–258)]

2. *Frontal bone.* Provides enclosure and protection of the brain.[24 (p. 170)]

3. *Frontal lobe.* Involved in personality, insight, and foresight; initiation of voluntary movements; written and spoken language.[6 (pp. 18–20)]

4. *Parietal bone.* Serves to enclose and protect the brain.[9 (p. 641), 24 (p. 170)]

5. *Parietal lobe.* The postcentral gyrus is the first somesthetic area; however, it also has a motor component. The association cortex allows for processing the significance of sensory data, including prior experience.[9 (p. 693), 12 (pp. 232–235)]

6. *Occipital lobe.* Involved in the higher order processing of visual information.[6 (pp. 21–22)]

7. *Superior temporal gyrus.* The primary auditory cortex.[1 (p. 161)]

8. *Occipital bone.* Forms the inferior and anterior walls of the posterior fossa.[4 (pp. 319–322)]

9. *Cerebellar hemisphere.* Involved with movements of the extremities and fine coordinated movements.[3 (p. 283), 12 (p. 175), 15 (pp. 633–634)]

10. *Middle temporal gyrus.* Functions as one of the multimodal association areas.[22 (p. 107)]

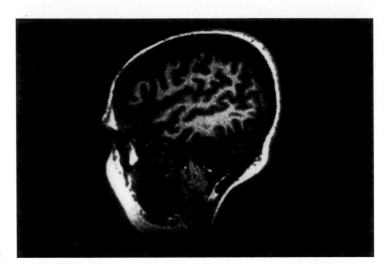

MRI

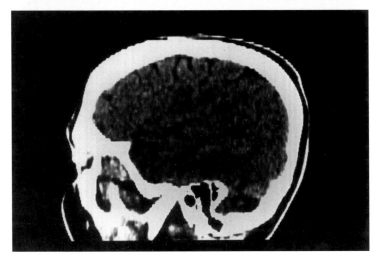

CT

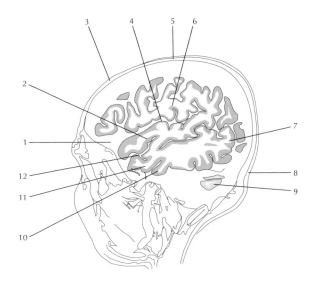

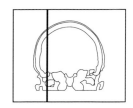

Sagittal 12

1. *Lesser wing of the sphenoid bone.* Forms part of the floor of the anterior cranial fossa.[9] (p. 676)

2. *Superior temporal gyrus.* The primary auditory cortex.[1] (p. 161)

3. *Frontal bone.* Provides enclosure and protection of the brain.[24] (p. 170)

4. *Auditory cortex.* Organized tonotopically for the processing of sound.[2] (pp. 182–184)

5. *Parietal bone.* Serves to enclose and protect the brain.[9] (p. 641), [24] (p. 170)

6. *Parietal lobe.* The postcentral gyrus is the first somesthetic area; however, it also has a motor component. The association cortex allows for processing the significance of sensory data, including prior experience.[9] (p. 693), [12] (pp. 232–235)

7. *Occipital lobe.* Involved in the higher order processing of visual information.[6] (pp. 21–22)

8. *Occipital bone.* Forms the inferior and anterior walls of the posterior fossa.[4] (pp. 319–322)

9. *Cerebellar hemisphere.* Involved with movements of the extremities and fine coordinated movements.[3] (p. 283), [12] (p. 175), [15] (pp. 633–634)

10. *Inferior temporal gyrus.* Involved in the analysis of the form and color of visual stimuli.[2] (pp. 154–157), [12] (p. 219)

11. *Middle temporal gyrus.* Functions as one of the multimodal association areas.[22] (p. 107)

12. *Superior temporal sulcus.* Serves to separate the superior and middle temporal gyri.[1] (p. 161)

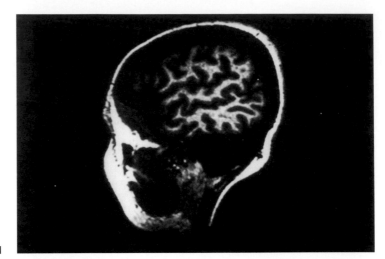

MRI

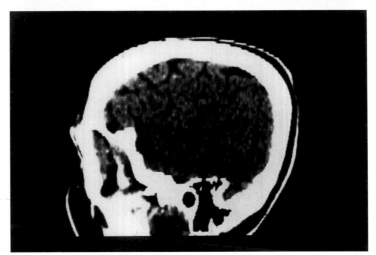

CT

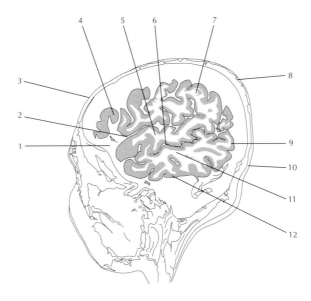

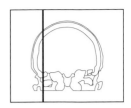

Sagittal 13

1. *Sphenoid bone.* The superior surface of the body is referred to as the sella turcica, which contains the pituitary gland.[9] (p. 645)

2. *Sylvian fissure (lateral sulcus or fissure).* Separates temporal lobe from frontal and parietal lobes.[19] (pp. 257–258)

3. *Frontal bone.* Provides enclosure and protection of the brain.[24] (p. 170)

4. *Frontal lobe.* Involved in personality, insight, and foresight; initiation of voluntary movements; written and spoken language.[6] (pp. 18–20)

5. *Superior temporal gyrus.* The primary auditory cortex.[1] (p. 161)

6. *Superior temporal sulcus.* Serves to separate the superior and middle temporal gyri.[1] (p. 161)

7. *Parietal lobe.* The postcentral gyrus is the first somesthetic area; however, it also has a motor component. The association cortex allows for processing the significance of sensory data, including prior experience.[9] (p. 693), [12] (pp. 232–235)

8. *Parietal bone.* Serves to enclose and protect the brain.[9] (p. 641), [24] (p. 170)

9. *Occipital lobe.* Involved in the higher order processing of visual information.[6] (pp. 21–22)

10. *Occipital bone.* Forms the inferior and anterior walls of the posterior fossa.[4] (pp. 319–322)

11. *Middle temporal gyrus.* Functions as one of the multimodal association areas.[22] (p. 107)

12. *Inferior temporal gyrus.* Involved in the analysis of the form and color of visual stimuli.[2] (pp. 154–157), [12] (p. 219)

Axial Views

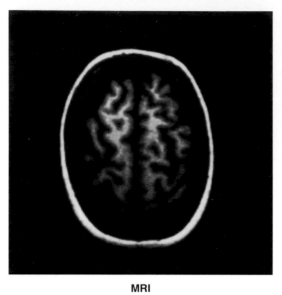

MRI

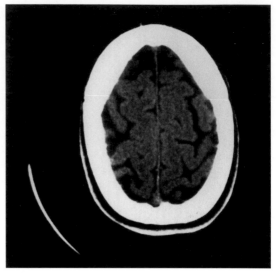

CT

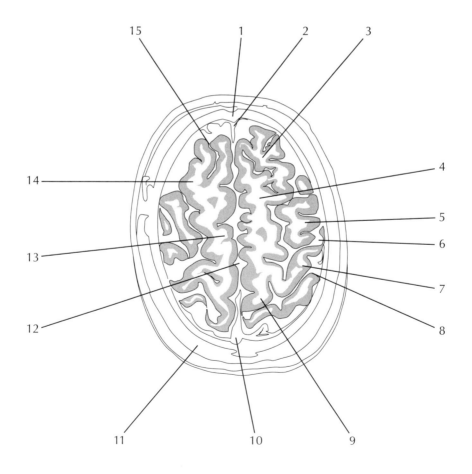

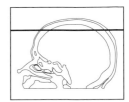

Axial 1

1. *Frontal bone.* Provides enclosure and protection of the brain.[24] (p. 170)
2. *Falx cerebri.* Separates the cerebral hemispheres.[19] (pp. 21, 491)
3. *Frontal lobe.* Involved in personality, insight, and foresight; initiation of voluntary movements; written and spoken language.[6] (pp. 18–20)
4. *Superior frontal gyrus.* Participates in the control and initiation of voluntary movements and is involved in personality, insight, and judgment.[6] (pp. 18–20), [18] (p. 674), [19] (p. 260)
5. *Precentral gyrus.* Location of the primary motor cortex.[1] (pp. 157, 326–327)
6. *Central sulcus.* Separates the primary motor cortex (frontal) from the primary somatosensory cortex (parietal).[19] (p. 257)
7. *Postcentral gyrus.* The area of the cortex associated with general sensory information.[6] (pp. 18–20)
8. *Postcentral sulcus.* Lies behind the postcentral gyrus.[6] (pp. 18–20)
9. *Superior parietal lobule.* Involved in sensory appreciation such as stereognosis, graphesthesia, and two-point discrimination.[3] (p. 404), [12] (pp. 17–18), [14] (p. 886)
10. *Superior sagittal sinus.* Drains blood from the brain and drains cerebrospinal fluid from the subarachnoid space.[11] (pp. 292, 439)
11. *Parietal bone.* Serves to enclose and protect the brain.[9] (p. 641), [24] (p. 170)
12. *Interhemispheric (longitudinal) fissure.* Separates the cerebral hemispheres.[12] (p. 218), [19] (p. 257)
13. *Paracentral lobule.* Medial extension of the precentral (motor) and postcentral (sensory) gyri.[6] (pp. 18–20)
14. *Middle frontal gyrus.* Participates in the control and initiation of voluntary movements; involved in personality, insight, and foresight.[6] (p. 18)
15. *Superior frontal sulcus.* Separates the superior frontal gyrus from the middle frontal gyrus.[12] (p. 219)

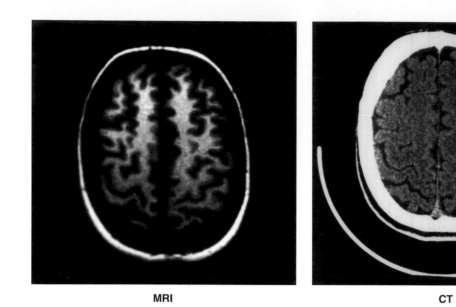

MRI

CT

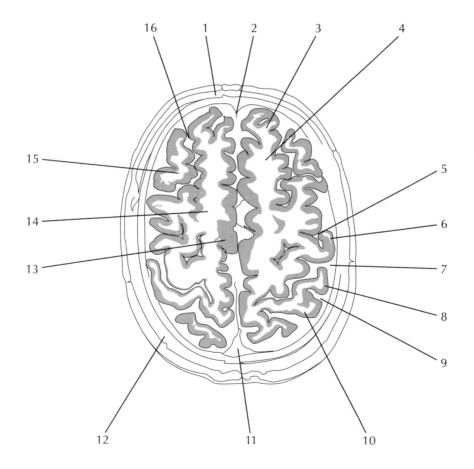

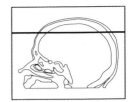

Axial 2

1. *Frontal bone.* Provides enclosure and protection of the brain.[24 (p. 170)]

2. *Falx cerebri.* Separates the cerebral hemispheres.[19 (pp. 21, 491)]

3. *Frontal lobe.* Involved in personality, insight, and foresight; initiation of voluntary movements; written and spoken language.[6 (pp. 18–20)]

4. *Superior frontal gyrus.* Participates in the control and initiation of voluntary movements and is involved in personality, insight, and judgment.[6 (pp. 18–20), 18 (p. 674), 19 (p. 260)]

5. *Precentral sulcus.* Anterior to the precentral gyrus.[6 (pp. 18–20)]

6. *Precentral gyrus.* Location of the primary motor cortex.[1 (pp. 157, 326–327)]

7. *Central sulcus.* Separates the primary motor cortex (frontal) from the primary somatosensory cortex (parietal).[19 (p. 257)]

8. *Postcentral gyrus.* The area of the cortex associated with general sensory information.[6 (pp. 18–20)]

9. *Postcentral sulcus.* Lies behind the postcentral gyrus.[6 (pp. 18–20)]

10. *Supramarginal gyrus.* Receives constructs of form, size, and body image from the somatosensory cortex; on the dominant side is involved in the comprehension of language.[3 (p. 409), 6 (pp. 18–20), 7 (pp. 405–407)]

11. *Superior sagittal sinus.* Drains blood from the brain and drains cerebrospinal fluid from the subarachnoid space.[11 (pp. 292, 439)]

12. *Parietal bone.* Serves to enclose and protect the brain.[9 (p. 641), 24 (p. 170)]

13. *Paracentral lobule.* Medial extension of the precentral (motor) and postcentral (sensory) gyri.[6 (pp. 18–20)]

14. *Centrum semiovale.* Superior radiation of the internal capsule.[13 (p. 86)]

15. *Middle frontal gyrus.* Participates in the control and initiation of voluntary movements; involved in personality, insight, and foresight.[6 (p. 18)]

16. *Superior frontal sulcus.* Separates the superior frontal gyrus from the middle frontal gyrus.[12 (p. 219)]

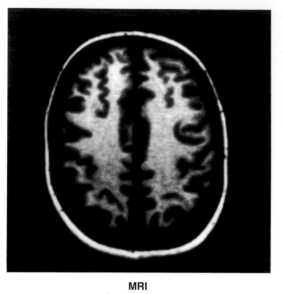

MRI

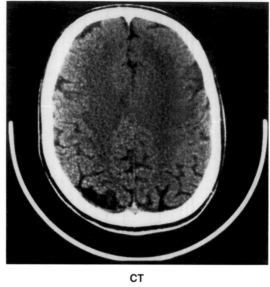

CT

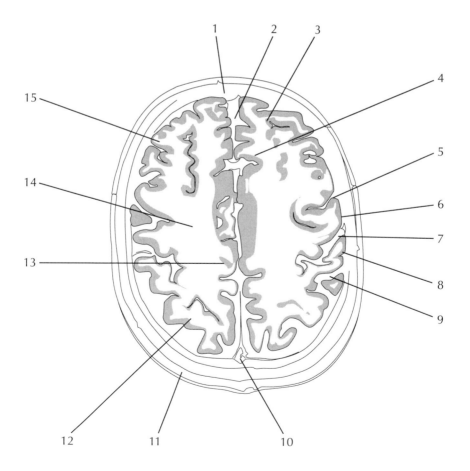

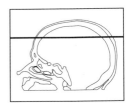

Axial 3

1. *Frontal bone.* Provides enclosure and protection of the brain.[24 (p. 170)]

2. *Interhemispheric (longitudinal) fissure.* Separates the cerebral hemispheres.[12 (p. 218), 19 (p. 257)]

3. *Frontal lobe.* Involved in personality, insight, and foresight; initiation of voluntary movements; written and spoken langauge.[6 (pp. 18–20)]

4. *Superior frontal gyrus.* Participates in the control and initiation of voluntary movements and is involved in personality, insight, and judgment.[6 (pp. 18–20), 18 (p. 674), 19 (p. 260)]

5. *Precentral sulcus.* Anterior to the precentral gyrus.[6 (pp. 18–20)]

6. *Precentral gyrus.* Location of the primary motor cortex.[1 (pp. 157, 326–327)]

7. *Central sulcus.* Separates the primary motor cortex (frontal) from the primary somatosensory cortex (parietal).[19 (p. 257)]

8. *Postcentral gyrus.* The area of the cortex associated with general sensory information.[6 (pp. 18–20)]

9. *Postcentral sulcus.* Lies behind the postcentral gyrus.[6 (pp. 18–20)]

10. *Superior sagittal sinus.* Drains blood from the brain and drains cerebrospinal fluid from the subarachnoid space.[11 (pp. 292, 439)]

11. *Parietal bone.* Serves to enclose and protect the brain.[9 (p. 641), 24 (pp. 170)]

12. *Inferior parietal lobule.* May involve written, visual, and auditory language integration.[3 (p. 409), 6 (p. 20), 14 (p. 848)]

13. *Paracentral lobule.* Medial extension of the precentral (motor) and postcentral (sensory) gyri.[6 (pp. 18–20)]

14. *Centrum semiovale.* Superior radiation of the internal capsule.[13 (p. 86)]

15. *Middle frontal gyrus.* Participates in the control and initiation of voluntary movements; involved in personality, insight, and foresight.[6 (p. 18)]

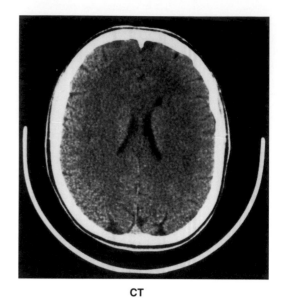

MRI

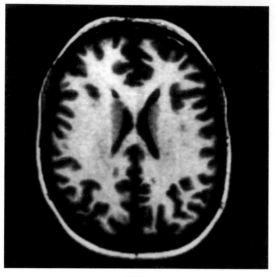

CT

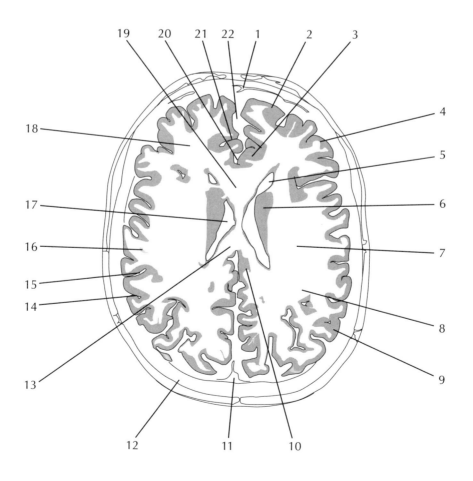

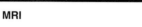

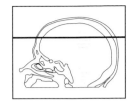

Axial 4

1. *Diploic space.* Loose osseous tissue between the two tables of the cranial bones.[14 (p. 450)]

2. *Superior frontal gyrus.* Participates in the control and initiation of voluntary movements and is involved in personality, insight, and judgment.[6 (pp. 18–20), 18 (p. 674), 19 (p. 260)]

3. *Cingulate gyrus (anterior).* Plays a role in emotional behavior, the autonomic nervous system, learning, and memory.[12 (p. 272), 18 (pp. 255, 674)]

4. *Middle frontal gyrus.* Participates in the control and initiation of voluntary movements; involved in personality, insight, and foresight.[6 (p. 18)]

5. *Anterior horn of the lateral ventricle.* Anterior ependymal-lined cavity.[1 (pp. 172–173), 11 (p. 283), 12 (pp. 253–256)]

6. *Caudate nucleus.* Involved in cognitive functions and movement.[6 (p. 304), 7 (p. 11), 12 (pp. 207–212), 15 (pp. 306–307), 18 (pp. 523–524)]

7. *Centrum semiovale.* Superior radiation of the internal capsule.[13 (p. 86)]

8. *Parietal lobe.* The postcentral gyrus is the first somesthetic area; however, it also has a motor component. The association cortex allows for processing the significance of sensory data, including prior experience.[9 (p. 693), 12 (pp. 232–235)]

9. *Angular gyrus.* On the dominant side is involved with the comprehension of language.[6 (pp. 18–20), 7 (pp. 405–407)]

10. *Cingulate gyrus (posterior).* Plays a role in emotional behavior, the autonomic nervous system, learning, and memory.[12 (p. 272), 18 (pp. 255, 674)]

11. *Superior sagittal sinus.* Drains blood from the brain and drains cerebrospinal fluid (CSF) from the subarachnoid space.[11 (pp. 292, 439)]

12. *Parietal bone.* Serves to enclose and protect the brain.[9 (p. 641), 24 (p. 170)]

13. *Splenium of corpus callosum.* Enlargement of corpus callosum posteriorly connecting the occipital lobes.[11 (pp. 244–244), 12 (p. 248), 19 (p. 269)]

14. *Postcentral sulcus.* Lies behind the postcentral gyrus.[6 (pp. 18–20)]

15. *Central sulcus.* Separates the primary motor cortex (frontal) from the primary somatosensory cortex (parietal).[19 (p. 257)]

16. *Precentral gyrus.* Location of the primary motor cortex.[1 (pp. 157, 326–327)]

17. *Lateral ventricle—body.* Ependymal-lined cavity filled with CSF.[11 (p. 183), 12 (pp. 253–256)]

18. *Frontal lobe.* Involved in personality, insight, and foresight; initiation of voluntary movements; written and spoken language.[6 (pp. 18–20)]

19. *Genu of corpus callosum.* Connects the frontal lobes.[2 (p. 51, 131), 12 (p. 248), 15 (p. 365), 19 (p. 269)]

20. *Callosal sulcus.* Separates the cingulate gyrus from the corpus callosum.[11 (p. 236)]

21. *Cingulate sulcus.* Separates the cingulate gyrus from the superior frontal gyrus.[19 (p. 261)]

22. *Interhemispheric (longitudinal) fissure.* Separates the cerebral hemispheres.[12 (p. 218), 19 (p. 257)]

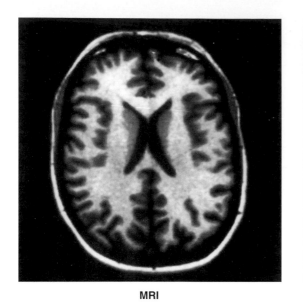

MRI

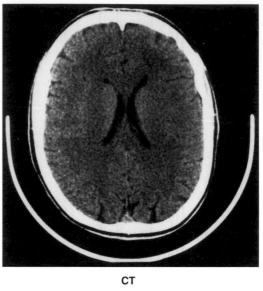

CT

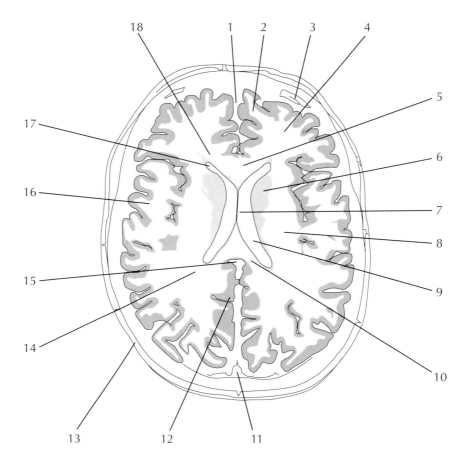

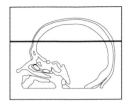

Axial 5

1. *Interhemispheric (longitudinal) fissure.* Separates the cerebral hemispheres.[12 (p. 218), 19 (p. 257)]

2. *Superior frontal gyrus.* Participates in the control and initiation of voluntary movements and is involved in personality, insight, and judgment.[6 (pp. 18–20), 18 (p. 674), 19 (p. 260)]

3. *Diploic space.* Loose osseous tissue between the two tables of the cranial bones.[14 (p. 450)]

4. *Frontal lobe.* Involved in personality, insight, and foresight; initiation of voluntary movements; written and spoken language.[6 (pp. 18–20)]

5. *Genu of the corpus callosum.* Connects the frontal lobes.[2 (pp. 51, 131), 12 (p. 248), 15 (p. 365), 19 (p. 269)]

6. *Caudate nucleus.* Involved in cognitive functions and movement.[6 (p. 304), 7 (p. 11), 12 (pp. 207–212), 15 (pp. 366–307), 18 (pp. 523–524)]

7. *Septum pellucidum.* Forms the medial wall of the body and anterior horns of the lateral ventricle.[2 (p. 384), 12 (pp. 249–250), 19 (p. 273)]

8. *Centrum semiovale.* Superior radiation of the internal capsule.[13 (p. 86)]

9. *Lateral ventricle—body.* Ependymal-lined C-shaped cavity of each hemisphere filled with cerebrospinal fluid (CSF).[11 (p. 183), 12 (pp. 253–256)]

10. *Splenium of corpus callosum.* Enlargement of corpus callosum posteriorly connecting the occipital lobe.[11 (pp. 244–245), 12 (p. 248), 19 (p. 269)]

11. *Superior sagittal sinus.* Drains blood from the brain and drains CSF from the subarachnoid space.[11 (pp. 292, 439)]

12. *Cingulate gyrus.* Plays a role in emotional behavior, the autonomic nervous system, learning, and memory.[12 (p. 272), 18 (pp. 255, 674)]

13. *Parietal bone.* Serves to enclose and protect the brain.[9 (p. 641), 24 (p. 170)]

14. *Forceps major (forceps occipitalis).* Interconnects the occipital lobes.[12 (p. 248)]

15. *Callosal sulcus.* Separates the cingulate gyrus from the corpus callosum.[11 (p. 236)]

16. *Temporal lobe.* Involved in emotions, visceral responses, learning, and memory.[6 (pp. 21–22)]

17. *Anterior horn of the lateral ventrical.* Anterior ependymal-lined cavity.[1 (pp. 172–173), 11 (p. 283), 12 (pp. 253–256)]

18. *Forceps minor (forceps frontalis).* Interconnects the frontal lobes.[12 (p. 248)]

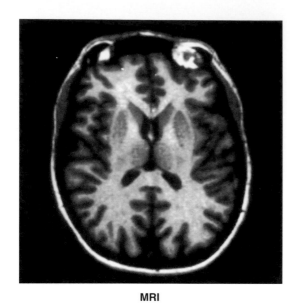

MRI

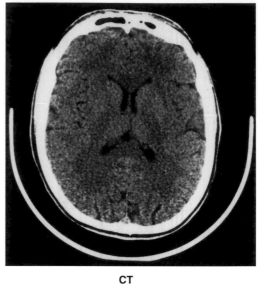

CT

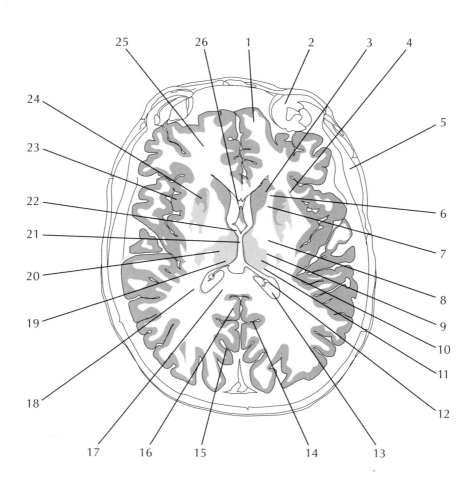

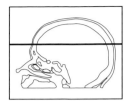

Axial 6

1. *Superior frontal gyrus.* Participates in the control and initiation of voluntary movements and is involved in personality, insight, and judgment.[6] (pp. 18–20), [18] (p. 674), [19] (p. 260)

2. *Orbital fat.* Provides cushioning and support of the eye.[25] (p. 188)

3. *Caudate nucleus.* Involved in cognitive functions and movement.[6] (p. 304), [7] (p. 11), [12] (pp. 207–211), [15] (pp. 306–307), [18] (pp. 523–524)

4. *Claustrum.* Involved in mediating visual attention.[11] (p. 244), [15] (p. 460)

5. *Temporalis muscle.* Assists in jaw closure.[8] (pp. 255–268)

6. *Internal capsule—anterior limb.* Connects subcortical nuclei with the cerebral cortex and the cerebral cortex with subcortical structures.[7] (p. 12), [11] (p. 249), [16] (p. 538)

7. *Internal capsule—genu.* Contains corticobulbar and corticoreticular connection fibers.[7] (p. 12), [11] (p. 249), [16] (p. 538)

8. *Internal capsule—posterior limb.* Contains fibers of general sensation.[7] (p. 12), [11] (p. 249), [16] (p. 538)

9. *Ventral lateral nucleus.* Conveys motor information from the cerebellum and globus pallidus to the precentral motor cortex.[3] (pp. 144–145), [22] (pp. 90–92)

10. *Ventral posterolateral nucleus.* Relays and modifies sensory signals from the face, retina, cochlea, taste receptors, and body.[3] (pp. 144–145), [22] (pp. 90–92)

11. *Thalamus.* Serves as the main relay center for the nervous system.[6] (p. 234), [20] (pp. 258–263)

12. *Choroid plexus of lateral ventricle.* Produces cerebrospinal fluid (CSF).[5] (p. 102), [14] (p. 1213)

13. *Lateral ventricle—atrium.* Ependymal-lined C-shaped cavity of each hemisphere filled with CSF.[11] (p. 183), [12] (pp. 253–256)

14. *Cingulate sulcus.* Separates the cingulate gyrus from the superior frontal gyrus.[19] (p. 261)

15. *Calcarine sulcus.* Marks the visual cortex.[11] (pp. 242, 260), [12] (pp. 217–218)

16. *Cingulate gyrus.* Plays a role in emotional behavior, the autonomic nervous system, learning, and memory.[12] (p. 272), [18] (pp. 255, 674)

17. *Splenium of the corpus callosum.* Enlargement of the corpus callosum posteriorly connecting the occipital lobes.[11] (pp. 244–245), [12] (p. 248), [19] (p. 269)

18. *Optic radiations.* Maintains a precise visuotopic organization from the lateral geniculate body to the primary visual cortex.[1] (p. 240)

19. *Pulvinar nucleus.* Along with the posterolateral and dorsolateral nuclei the pulvinar nucleus forms the multimodal functional division of the thalamic nuclei.[3] (pp. 144–145), [22] (pp. 90–92)

20. *Lateral dorsal nucleus.* Major relay nuclei for the limbic system circuits.[1] (p. 444)

21. *Third ventricle.* Transmits CSF from the lateral ventricles to the fourth ventricle.[5] (p. 103)

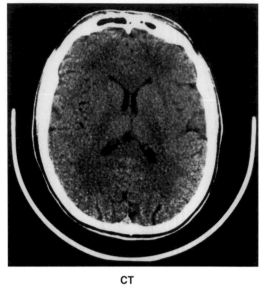

MRI

CT

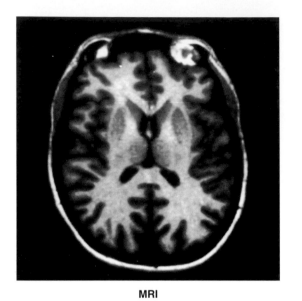

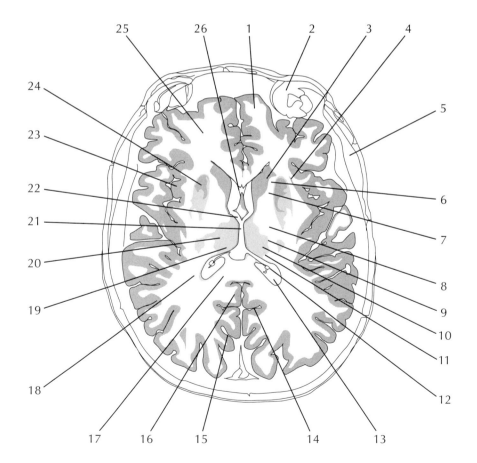

22. *Columns of fornix—anterior.* Part of the myelinated pathway connecting the hippocampus with subcortical structures.[11] (p. 276), 12 (pp. 268–269), 19 (p. 269)

23. *Insular cortex (Island of Reil).* Associated with visceral functions, and anteriorly contains the cortical gustatory (taste) area.[2] (p. 196), 12 (pp. 209–213), 19 (p. 294)

24. *Putamen.* Involved in motor function.[6] (p. 304), 7 (p. 11)

25. *Frontal lobe.* Involved in personality, insight, and foresight; initiation of voluntary movements; written and spoken language.[6] (pp. 18–20)

26. *Septum pellucidum.* Forms the medial wall of the body and anterior horns of the lateral ventricle.[2] (p. 384), 12 (pp. 249–250), 19 (p. 273)

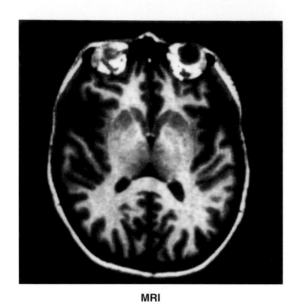

MRI

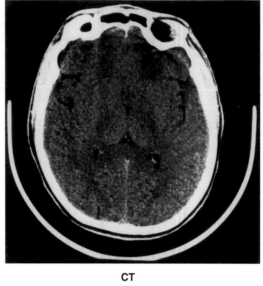

CT

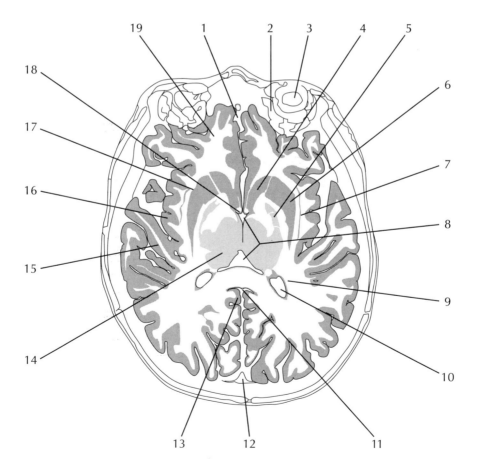

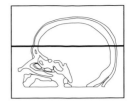

Axial 7

1. *Interhemispheric (longitudinal) fissure.* Separates the cerebral hemispheres.[12] (p. 218), [19] (p. 257)

2. *Orbital fat.* Provides cushioning and support of the eye.[25] (p. 188)

3. *Globe.* Complex structure for vision.[8] (pp. 380–384), [25] (p. 188)

4. *Caudate nucleus.* Involved in cognitive functions and movement.[6] (p. 304), [7] (p. 11), [12] (pp. 207–212), [15] (pp. 306–307), [18] (pp. 523–524)

5. *Globus pallidus.* Involved in the control of movement.[6] (p. 306), [7] (p. 11), [20] (pp. 276–277)

6. *Putamen.* Involved in motor function.[6] (p. 304), [7] (p. 11)

7. *Claustrum.* Involved in mediating visual attention.[11] (p. 244), [15] (p. 460)

8. *Third ventricle.* Transmits cerebrospinal fluid (CSF) from the lateral ventricles to the fourth ventricle.[5] (p. 103)

9. *Optic radiations.* Maintains a precise visutopic organization from the lateral geniculate body to the primary visual cortex.[1] (p. 240)

10. *Posterior horn of the lateral ventricle.* Ependymal-lined cavity extending into the occipital lobe.[11] (pp. 242, 246)

11. *Callosal sulcus.* Separates the cingulate gyrus from the corpus callosum.[11] (p. 236)

12. *Superior sagittal sinus.* Drains blood from the brain and drains CSF from the subarachnoid space.[11] (pp. 292, 439)

13. *Cingulate gyrus.* Plays a role in emotional behavior, the autonomic nervous system, learning, and memory.[12] (p. 272), [18] (pp. 255, 674)

14. *Thalamus.* Serves as the main relay center for the nervous system.[6] (p. 234), [20] (pp. 258–263)

15. *Temporal lobe.* Involved in emotions, visceral responses, learning, and memory.[6] (pp. 21–22)

16. *Insular cortex (island of Reil).* Associated with visceral functions and anteriorly contains the cortical gustatory (taste) area.[2] (p. 196), [12] (pp. 209–213), [19] (p. 294)

17. *Basal ganglia.* Involved in both cognitive and motor functions.[6] (p. 304), [7] (p. 11)

18. *Fornix.* Efferent tract of the hippocampus projecting to the mamillary bodies.[11] (p. 276), [12] (pp. 268–269), [19] (p. 269)

19. *Frontal lobe.* Consists of four functional areas and involved in personality, insight, and foresight; initiation of voluntary movements; written and spoken language.[6] (pp. 18–20)

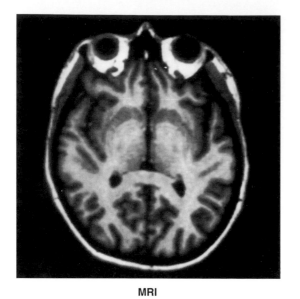

MRI

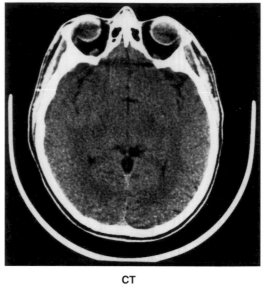

CT

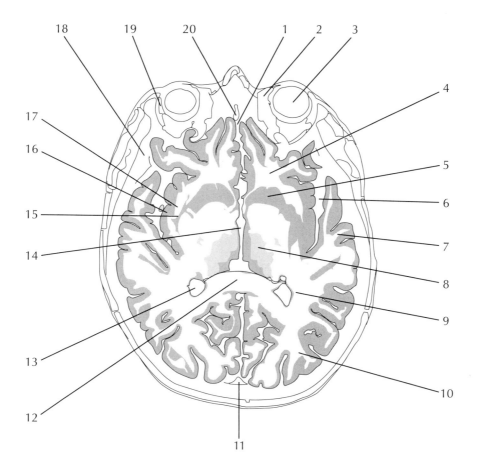

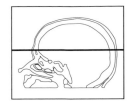

Axial 8

1. *Interhemispheric (longitudinal) fissure.* Separates the cerebral hemispheres.[12] (p. 218), [19] (p. 257)

2. *Orbital fat.* Provides cushioning and support of the eye.[25] (p. 188)

3. *Globe.* Complex structure for vision.[8] (pp. 380–384), [25] (p. 188)

4. *Frontal lobe.* Involved in personality, insight and foresight; initiation of voluntary movements; written and spoken language.[6] (pp. 18–20)

5. *Putamen.* Involved in motor function.[6] (p. 304), [7] (p. 11)

6. *Sylvian fissure (lateral sulcus or fissure).* Separates temporal lobe from frontal and parietal lobes.[19] (pp. 257–258)

7. *Temporal lobe.* Involved in emotions, visceral responses, learning, and memory.[6] (pp. 21–22)

8. *Thalamus.* Serves as the main relay center for the nervous system.[6] (p. 234), [20] (pp. 258–263)

9. *Optic radiations.* Maintains a precise visuotopic organization from the lateral geniculate body to the primary visual cortex.[1] (p. 240)

10. *Occipital lobe.* Involved in the higher order processing of visual information.[6] (pp. 21–22)

11. *Superior sagittal sinus.* Drains blood from the brain and drains cerebrospinal fluid (CSF) from the subarachnoid space.[11] (pp. 292, 439)

12. *Corpus callosum.* Interconnects the cerebral hemispheres.[2] (p.131), [12] (p. 248), [16] (p. 33), [21] (4)

13. *Posterior horn of the lateral ventricle.* Ependymal-lined cavity extending into the occipital lobe.[11] (pp. 242, 260)

14. *Third ventricle.* Transmits CSF from the lateral ventricles to the fourth ventricle.[5] (p. 103)

15. *Claustrum.* Involved in mediating visual attention.[11] (p. 244), [15] (p. 460)

16. *Insular cortex (island of Reil).* Associated with visceral functions, and anteriorly contains the cortical gustatory (taste) area.[2] (p. 196), [12] (pp. 209–213), [19] (p. 294)

17. *Extreme capsule.* Contains corticocortical association fibers.[2] (p. 276), [12] (p. 209)

18. *Frontal bone.* Provides enclosure and protection of the brain.[24] (p. 170)

19. *Lacrimal gland.* Produces lacrimal fluid (tears).[9] (pp. 711–712)

20. *Crista galli.* Serves as an attachment for the falx cerebri.[22] (p. 124)

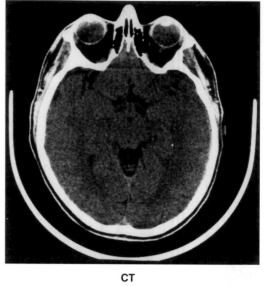

MRI

CT

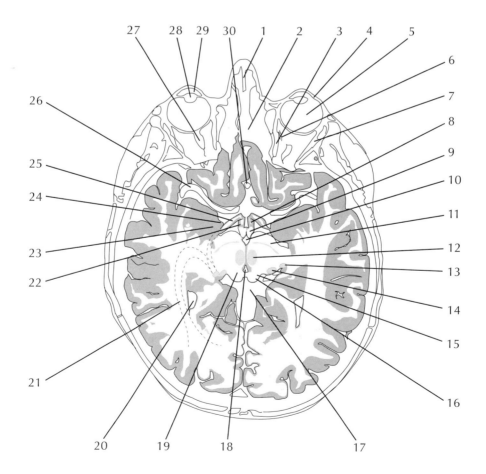

27 28 29 30 1 2 3 4 5

26

25

24

23

22

21

6

7

8

9

10

11

12

13

14

15

16

20 19 18 17

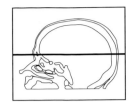

Axial 9

1. *Vomer.* A bony structure forming the back and lower part of the nasal septum.[8] (p. 123)

2. *Ethmoid air cells.* Act as resonators to the voice.[23] (pp. 734–736)

3. *Superior oblique muscle.* Depresses the medially rotated eye, rotates medially, and abducts the eyeball.[9] (pp. 715–717)

4. *Sclera.* Forms the "white" of the eye.[9] (pp. 705–708)

5. *Globe.* Complex structure for vision.[8] (pp. 380–384), [25] (p. 188)

6. *Superior opthalamic vein.* Anastomosis with the facial vein and allows blood to flow in either direction, since it has no valves.[9] (p. 719)

7. *Lateral rectus muscle.* Rotates the eye so that the cornea is directed laterally.[9] (p. 715), [25] (p. 189)

8. *Tuber cinereum.* A swelling that has most of the hypothalamic nuclei that regulate the release of the anterior pituitary hormones.[2] (p. 350), [12] (p. 196)

9. *Mamillary body.* Receives hippocampal input.[1] (p. 386), [2] (pp. 367–368, 381, 392)

10. *Interpeduncular cistern.* Enlargement of the subarachnoid space on the anterior brainstem.[7] (p. 69), [11] (p. 443)

11. *Cerebral peduncle.* Forms both sides of the midbrain, excluding the tectum.[2] (p. 226), [12] (p. 108)

12. *Red nucleus.* Relays impulses from the cerebral and cerebellar cortex to the spinal cord.[1] (p. 353), [2] (pp. 225–226, 250), [16] (pp. 435–436)

13. *Lateral geniculate body.* The principal thalamic relay nucleus for the visual system.[1] (p. 444), [2] (pp. 154–160)

14. *Medial geniculate body (nucleus).* Primary source of fibers ending in the auditory cortex.[1] (p. 444), [3] (p. 193), [12] (p. 236), [15] (p. 181)

15. *Pretectal area.* Involved in a reflex pathway for pupillary light response and cortical control of eye movement.[1] (p. 411), [12] (p. 112)

16. *Superior colliculus.* Receives visual signals directly from the retina or indirectly from the visual cortex and is essential for rapid eye movements.[1] (pp. 245–246, 412)

17. *Quadrigeminal plate cistern (retropulvinar cistern).* Enlarged subarachnoid space.[10] (pp. 120–121)

18. *Cerebral aqueduct (aqueduct of Sylvius).* Connects the third and fourth ventricles.[2] (p. 22), [11] (p. 213)

19. *Superior cerebellar peduncle.* Connects the cerebellum to the midbrain.[2] (pp. 242, 249), [11] (p. 13), [12] (p. 104–105), [20] (p. 326)

20. *Posterior horn of the lateral ventricle.* Ependymal lined cavity extending into the occipital lobe.[11] (pp. 242, 260)

21. *Optic radiation.* Maintains a precise visuotopic organization from the lateral geniculate body to the primary visual cortex.[1] (p. 240)

22. *Hypothalamus.* Regulates the autonomic nervous system and also controls pituitary function.[3] (pp. 421–424)

23. *Uncus of temporal lobe.* Anterior part of

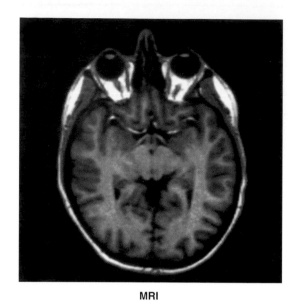

MRI

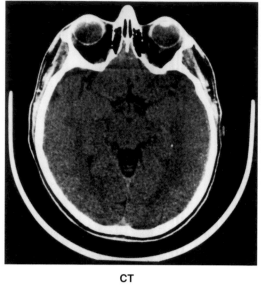

CT

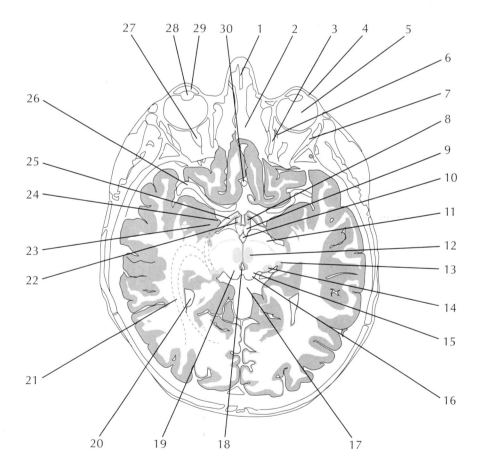

the parahippocampal gyrus, used as an anatomic landmark.[2 (pp. 200–202), 6 (p. 21–22)]

24. *Anterior perforated substance.* Contains the olfactory tubercle.[2 (pp. 200–202)]

25. *Optic tract.* Transmission of visual impulses from the retina.[15 (p. 424), 19 (p. 399)]

26. *Middle cerebral artery.* Provides vascular supply to the insular cortex and lateral surface of the hemisphere.[1 (p. 186), 10 (pp. 207–211)]

27. *Optic nerve (cranial nerve II).* Nerve of sight.[7 (pp. 221, 227)]

28. *Lens.* Completes the refraction of entering light.[24 (pp. 283–287)]

29. *Cornea.* Responsible for refraction of the light that enters the eye.[9 (p. 714)]

30. *Anterior cerebral artery.* Supplies the orbital and medial frontal lobe as well as the medial parietal lobe.[7 (p. 59), 10 (p. 191)]

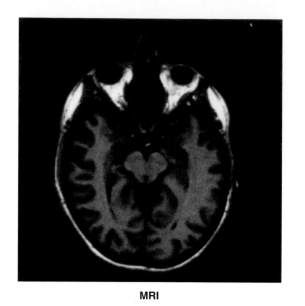

MRI

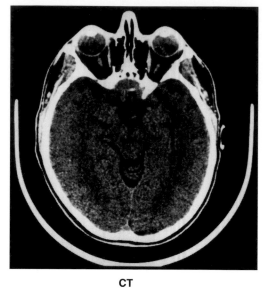

CT

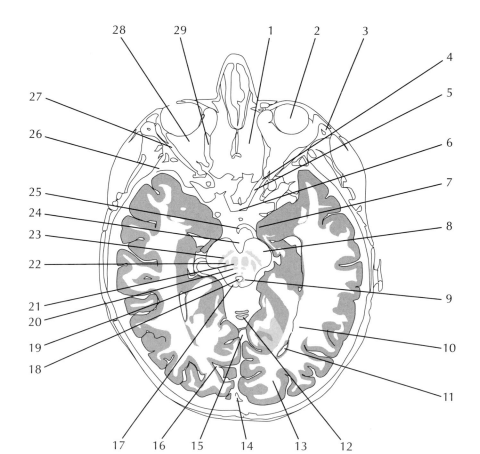

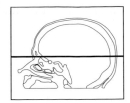

Axial 10

1. *Ethmoid air cells.* Act as resonators to the voice.[23] (pp. 734–736)

2. *Globe.* Complex structure for vision.[8] (pp. 380–384), [25] (p. 188)

3. *Zygomatic process of frontal bone.* The lateral aspect of the superior orbit.[4] (p. 333)

4. *Optic canal.* Transversed by the optic nerve (cranial-nerve II) and the ophthalmic arteries.[9] (p. 679)

5. *Optic nerve.* Nerve of sight.[7] (pp. 221, 227)

6. *Optic chiasm.* Convergence of the optic nerves.[2] (p. 143), [11] (p. 227)

7. *Uncus of temporal lobe.* Anterior part of the parahippocampal gyrus, used as an anatomic landmark.[2] (pp. 200–202), [6] (pp. 21–22)

8. *Cerebral peduncle.* Forms both sides of the midbrain, excluding the tectum.[2] (p. 226), [12] (p. 108)

9. *Periaqueductal gray matter.* Plays a role in endogenous pain suppression and contains high concentrations of opioid peptides (endorphins).[1] (p. 220), [2] (p. 68)

10. *Optic radiation.* Maintains precise visuotopic organization from the lateral geniculate body to the primary visual cortex.[1] (p. 240)

11. *Lateral ventricle—occipital pole.* Ependymal-lined C-shaped cavity of each hemisphere filled with cerebrospinal fluid (CSF).[11] (p. 183), [12] (pp. 253–256)

12. *Cerebellar vermis.* Regulates and coordinates axial and girdle musculature.[3] (p. 282), [7] (p. 290)

13. *Occipital lobe.* Involved in the higher order processing of visual information.[6] (pp. 21–22)

14. *Superior sagittal sinus.* Drains blood from the brain and drains CSF from the subarachnoid space.[11] (pp. 292, 439)

15. *Straight venous sinus.* Provides cerebral venous drainage.[7] (p. 61), [22] (pp. 440–441)

16. *Calcarine sulcus.* Marks the visual cortex.[1] (p. 242, 260), [3] (p. 217–218)

17. *Superior colliculus.* Receives visual signals directly from the retina or indirectly from the visual cortex and is essential for rapid eye movements.[1] (pp. 245–246, 412)

18. *Cerebral aqueduct.* Connects the third and fourth ventricles.[2] (p. 22), [11] (p. 213)

19. *Oculomotor nucleus.* Contains the motor neurons of the oculomotor nerve.[2] (pp. 322–323)

20. *Medial longitudinal fasciculus.* Brainstem pathway essential for the control of eye movements.[2] (p. 173)

21. *Red nucleus.* Relays impulses from the cerebral and cerebellar cortex to the spinal cord.[1] (p. 353), [2] (pp. 225–226, 250), [16] (pp. 435–436)

22. *Medial lemniscus.* Transmits touch and proprioception for the contralateral side of the body.[1] (pp. 203–206)

23. *Substantia nigra.* Has a regulatory effect on the neostriatum through the action of dopamine.[12] (pp. 114–115), [20] (pp. 276–277)

24. *Interpeduncular fossa.* Subarachnoid space between the cerebral peduncles.[10] (pp. 116–117)

25. *Posterior cerebral artery.* Supplies the

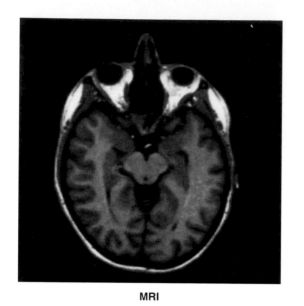

MRI

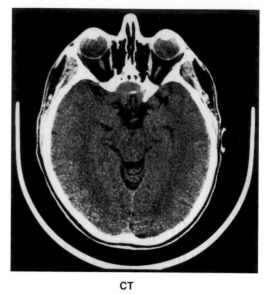

CT

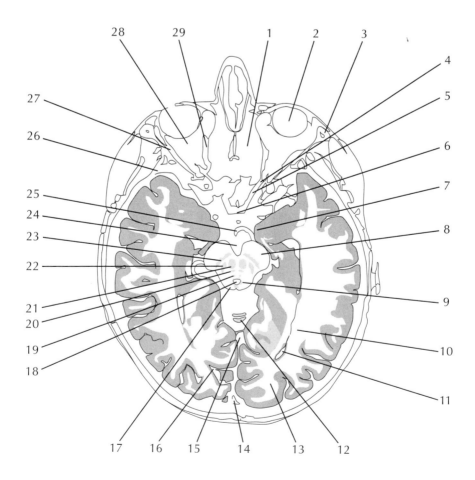

inferior and medial surface of the parietal and temporal lobes.[1 (p. 186), 10 (pp. 248–251)]

26. *Sphenoid bone.*   The superior surface of the body is referred to as the sella turcica, which contains the pituitary gland.[9 (p. 645)]

27. *Lateral rectus muscle.*   Rotates the eye so that the cornea is directed laterally.[9 (p. 715), 25 (p. 189)]

28. *Orbital fat.*   Provides cushioning and support of the eye.[25 (p. 188)]

29. *Medial rectus muscle.*   Rotates the eye so that the cornea is directed medially.[9 (p. 715), 25 (p. 189)]

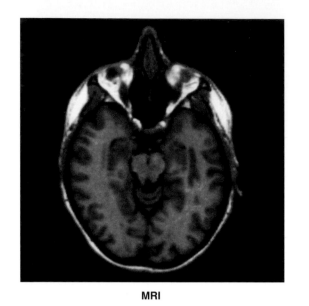

MRI

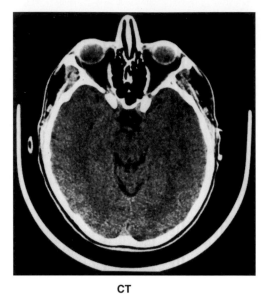

CT

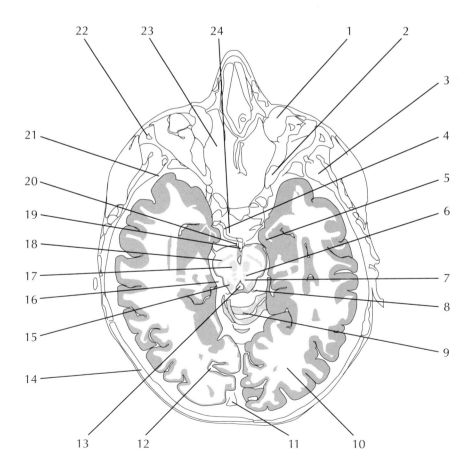

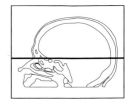

Axial 11

1. *Orbital fat.* Provides cushioning and support of the eye.[25] (p. 188)

2. *Inferior rectus muscle.* Serves to depress, adduct, and laterally rotate the eye.[9] (pp. 715—717)

3. *Temporalis muscle.* Assists in jaw closure.[8](pp. 255—268)

4. *Posterior communicating artery.* Arises from the internal carotid artery and joins the posterior cerebral artery.[1] (p. 179), [10] (p. 178)

5. *Uncus of temporal lobe.* Anterior part of the parahippocampal gyrus, used as an anatomic landmark.[2] (pp. 200–202), [6] (pp. 21–22)

6. *Medial longitudinal fasciculus.* Brainstem pathway essential for the control of eye movements.[2] (p. 173)

7. *Trochlear nucleus.* Contains the motor neurons of the trochlear nerve. Allows for movement of the eye down and out.[1] (p. 41), [2] (pp. 322–333)

8. *Trochlear nerve (cranial nerve IV).* Innervates the superior oblique muscle for movement of the eye down and out.[1] (p. 410)

9. *Cerebellar vermis.* Regulates and coordinates axial and girdle musculature.[3] (p. 282), [7] (p. 290)

10. *Occipital lobe.* Involved in the higher order processing of visual information.[6] (pp. 21–22)

11. *Superior sagittal sinus.* Drains blood from the brain and drains cerebrospinal fluid from the subarachnoid space.[11] (pp. 292, 439)

12. *Calcarine sulcus.* Marks the visual cortex.[11] (pp. 242, 260), [12] (pp. 217–218)

13. *Cerebral aqueduct (aqueduct of Sylvius).* Connects the third and fourth ventricles.[2] (p. 22), [11] (p. 213)

14. *Occipital bone.* Forms the inferior and anterior walls of the posterior fossa.[4] (pp. 319–322)

15. *Lateral lemniscus.* Transmits auditory information.[1] (p. 264), [3] (p. 199)

16. *Ambient cistern.* Envelopes the mesencephalon.[5] (p. 116)

17. *Red nucleus.* Relays impulses from the cerebral and cerebellar cortex to the spinal cord.[1] (p. 353), [2] (pp. 225–226, 250), [16] (pp. 435–436)

18. *Substantia nigra.* Has a regulatory effect on the neostriatum through the action of dopamine.[12] (pp. 114–115), [20] (pp. 276–277)

19. *Interpeduncular cistern.* Enlargement of the subarachnoid space on the anterior brainstem.[7] (p. 69), [11] (p. 443)

20. *Oculomotor nerve.* Innervates four of the six extraocular muscles as well as the levator palpebrae.[2] (pp. 322–333), [25] (p. 189)

21. *Sphenoid bone.* The superior surface of the body is referred to as the sella turcica, which contains the pituitary gland.[9] (p. 645)

22. *Frontal process of zygomatic bone.* Forms the lateral margin of the orbit.[9] (p. 655)

23. *Ethmoid air cells.* Act as resonators to the voice.[23] (pp. 734–736)

24. *Crural cistern.* Subarachnoid space through which the posterior communicating artery passes.[10] (p. 117)

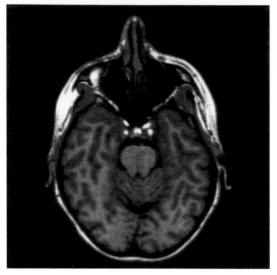

MRI

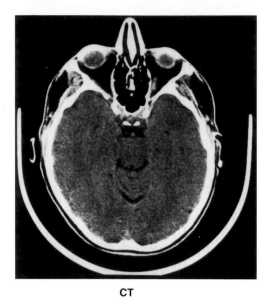

CT

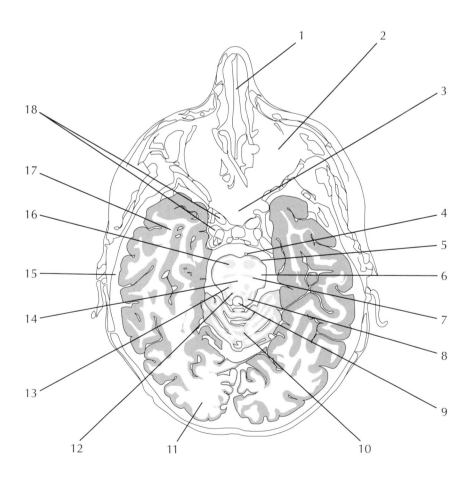

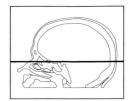

Axial 12

1. *Nasal septum.* Separates the right and left nasal fossae (cavities).[14 (p. 1402)]

2. *Maxillary sinus.* Acts as a resonator to the voice.[23 (pp. 734–736)]

3. *Sphenoid sinus.* Acts as a resonator to the voice.[23 (734–736)]

4. *Basilar artery.* Blood supply to upper medulla, pons, cerebellum, inner ear, occipital lobe, and part of the temporal lobe.[15 (p. 1042)]

5. *Pons.* Contains neural circuits that transmit information between the spinal cord and higher brain regions. Regulates levels of arousal, blood pressure, and respiration.[2 (p. 9), 11 (p. 181)]

6. *Middle cerebellar peduncle.* Connects cerebellum to pons, relaying input from the contralateral cerebral cortex to the lateral lobe of the cerebellum.[2 (pp. 242, 249), 11 (p. 13), 12 (pp. 104–105)]

7. *Medial lemniscus.* Transmits touch and proprioception for the contralateral side of the body.[1 (pp. 203–206)]

8. *Superior cerebellar peduncle.* Connects the cerebellum to the midbrain.[2 (p. 242, 249), 11 (p. 13), 12 (pp. 104–105), 20 (p. 326)]

9. *Fourth ventricle.* Cavity filled with cerebrospinal fluid.[7 (p. 70), 13 (p. 97)]

10. *Cerebellar vermis.* Regulates and coordinates axial and girdle musculature.[3 (p. 282), 7 (p. 290)]

11. *Occipital lobe.* Involved in the higher order of processing of visual information.[6 (pp. 21–22)]

12. *Medial longitudinal fasciculus.* Brainstem pathway essential for the control of eye movements.[2 (p. 173)]

13. *Trigeminal nucleus.* Contains motor neurons with fibers in the trigeminal nerve (cranial nerve V) with principal innervation to the muscles of mastication.[2 (pp. 322–333)]

14. *Reticular formation.* Involved in sleep and arousal activities, the motor system, and regulation of visceral activities.[2 (p. 229), 12 (p. 148)]

15. *Temporal bone.* Contains the organs of hearing.[14 (p. 219)]

16. *Pyramidal (corticospinal) tract.* Pathway for the control of contralateral voluntary motor activity for the body.[2 (pp. 208–210), 3 (p. 193), 12 (p. 148)]

17. *Temporal lobe.* Involved in emotions, visceral responses, learning, and memory.[6 (pp. 21–22)]

18. *Internal carotid artery.* Supplies eye and associated tissues, pituitary gland, and anterior portion of the brain.[4 (p. 686)]

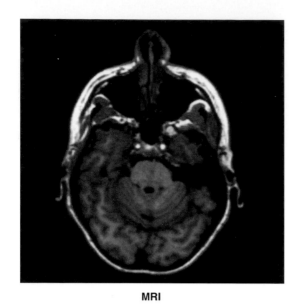

MRI

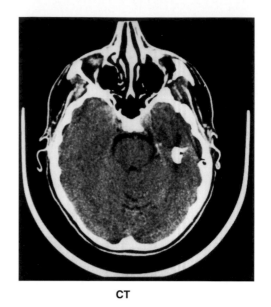

CT

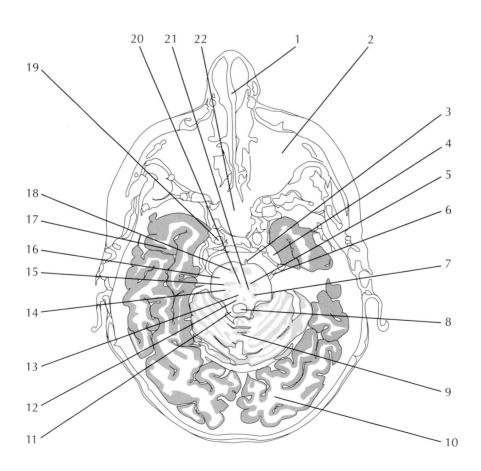

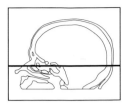

Axial 13

1. *Nasal septum.* Separates the right and left nasal fossae (cavities).[14] (p. 1402)

2. *Maxillary sinus.* Acts as a resonator to the voice.[23] (pp. 734–736)

3. *Abducens nerve (cranial nerve VI).* Lateral rectus muscle innervation (abduction).[1] (p. 104)

4. *Meckel's cave (trigeminal cave).* Location of the proximal trigeminal ganglion and the roots of the trigeminal nerve.[4] (p. 1045), [12] (p. 382)

5. *Medial lemniscus.* Transmits touch and proprioception for the contralateral side of the body.[1] (pp. 203–206)

6. *Trigeminal nerve (cranial nerve V).* Provides sensation to the face, most of the scalp, and the teeth, as well as the nasal and oral cavities. Also provides motor innervation to muscles of mastication.[1] (p. 404), [4] (p. 1059)

7. *Trigeminal nucleus.* Contains motor neurons with fibers in the trigeminal nerve (cranial nerve V) with principal innervation to the muscles of mastication.[2] (pp. 322–333)

8. *Fourth ventricle.* Cavity filled with cerebrospinal fluid.[7] (p. 70), [13] (p. 97)

9. *Cerebellar vermis.* Regulates and coordinates axial and girdle musculature.[3] (p. 282), [7] (p. 290)

10. *Occipital lobe.* Involved in the higher order processing of visual information.[6] (pp. 21–22)

11. *Superior cerebellar peduncle.* Connects the cerebellum to the midbrain.[2] (pp. 242, 249), [11] (p. 13), [12] (pp. 104–105), [20] (p. 326)

12. *Medial longitudinal fasciculus.* Brainstem pathway essential for the control of eye movements.[2] (p. 173)

13. *Reticular formation (of pons).* Involved in sleep and arousal activities, the motor system, and regulation of visceral activities.[2] (p. 229), [12] (p. 148)

14. *Lateral spinothalamic tract.* Transmits pain and temperature from the contralateral side of the body.[2] (p. 125), [3] (p. 193)

15. *Ventral spinothalamic tract.* Transmits contralateral light touch from the body.[2] (p. 125), [3] (p. 193), [20] (pp. 180–181)

16. *Middle cerebellar peduncle.* Connects cerebellum to pons, relaying input from the contralateral cerebral cortex to the lateral lobe of the cerebellum.[2] (pp. 242, 249), [11] (p. 13), [12] (pp. 104–105)

17. *Temporal lobe.* Involved in emotions, visceral responses, learning, and memory.[6] (pp. 21–22)

18. *Pyramidal tract.* Pathway for the control of contralateral voluntary motor activity for the body.[2] (pp. 208–210), [3] (p. 193), [12] (p. 148)

19. *Internal carotid artery.* Supplies eye and associated tissues, pituitary gland, and anterior portion of the brain.[4] (p. 686)

20. *Raphe nuclei.* Involved in the general behavioral state, perception of pain, and the sleep-wake cycle.[1] (pp. 220, 464), [12] (p. 149), [13] (p. 231)

21. *Dorsal trigeminothalamic tract.* Transmits ipsilateral touch and pressure sensations from the face.[2] (p. 307), [3] (p. 193)

22. *Sphenoid sinus.* Acts as a resonator to the voice.[23] (pp. 734–736)

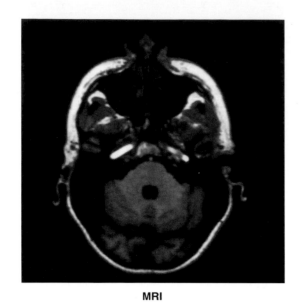

MRI

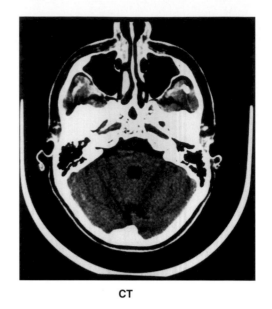

CT

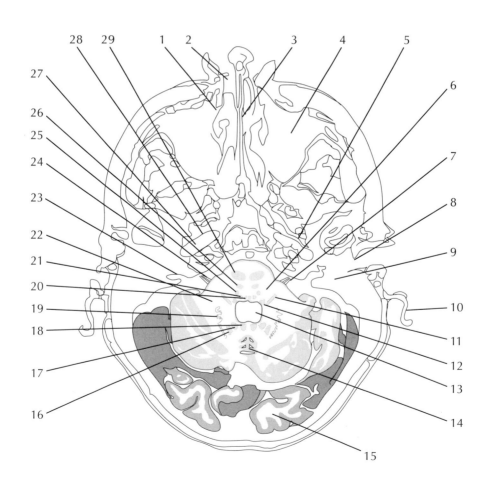

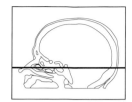

Axial 14

1. *Nasolacrimal canal.* Contains the naso-lacrimal duct.[14] [(p. 251)]
2. *Nasal cavity.* Aids in warming and moistening inspired air.[4] [(p. 1142)]
3. *Nasal septum.* Separates the right and left nasal fossae (cavities).[14] [(p. 1402)]
4. *Maxillary sinus.* Acts as a resonator to the voice.[23] [(pp. 734–736)]
5. *Eustachian tube (auditory tube, pharyngotympanic tube).* Equalizes air pressure, allowing free movement of the tympanic membrane.[9] [(p. 772)], [14] [(p. 1625)]
6. *Inferior cerebellar peduncle.* Connects the cerebellum to the medulla and is important in maintaining equilibrium.[2] [(pp. 242, 249)], [11] [(p. 13)], [12] [(pp. 104–105)]
7. *Auditory nerve (vestibulocochlear nerve, cranial nerve VIII).* Carries somatosensory impulses from specialized inner ear receptors.[13] [(pp. 245–246)]
8. *External auditory (acoustic) meatus.* Essential for the effective mechanical responses of the tympanic membrane.[4] [(p. 1192)]
9. *Temporal bone.* Contains the organs of hearing.[14] [(p. 219)]
10. *Auricle.* Collects air vibrations.[14] [(p. 167)]
11. *Auditory nucleus (VIII) (cochlear).* Important in localizing and recognizing patterns of sound.[2] [(pp. 166–167)]
12. *Auditory nucleus (VIII) (vestibular).* Transmits information involved with equilibrium.[2] [(p. 167)], [3] [(p. 199)]
13. *Fourth ventricle.* Cavity filled with cerebrospinal fluid.[7] [(p. 70)], [13] [(p. 97)]
14. *Cerebellar vermis.* Regulates and coordinates axial and girdle musculature.[3] [(p. 282)], [7] [(p. 290)]
15. *Occipital lobe.* Involved in the higher order processing of visual information.[6] [(pp. 21–22)]
16. *Emboliform nucleus.* Involved in the neural circuitry of the cerebellum.[2] [(p. 242)], [6] [(pp. 350—353)], [20] [(pp. 322–329)]
17. *Globose nucleus.* Involved in the neural circuitry of the cerebellum.[2] [(p. 242)], [6] [(pp. 350–353)], [20] [(pp. 322–329)]
18. *Fastigial nucleus.* Affects postural and proximal limb movement.[1] [(pp. 352–354)]
19. *Dentate nucleus.* Plays a role in somatic motor activity.[1] [(pp. 353–354)]
20. *Medial longitudinal fasciculus.* Brainstem pathway essential for the control of eye movements.[2] [(p. 173)]
21. *Abducens nucleus (VI).* Motor neurons of the abducens nerve.[1] [(p. 404)], [2] [(pp. 322–330)]
22. *Middle cerebellar peduncle.* Connects cerebellum to pons, relaying input from the contralateral cerebral cortex to the lateral lobe of the cerebellum.[2] [(pp. 242, 249)], [11] [(p. 13)], [12] [(pp. 104–105)]
23. *Internal auditory canal.* Transmits the facial nerve (VII), the auditory nerve (VIII), the nervous intermedius, and the labyrinthine vessels.[9] [(p. 681)]
24. *Facial nerve (cranial nerve VII).* Consists

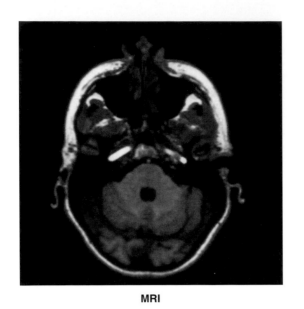

MRI

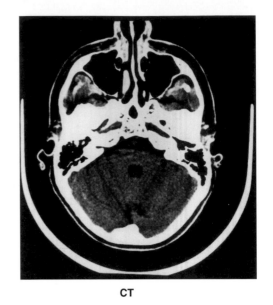

CT

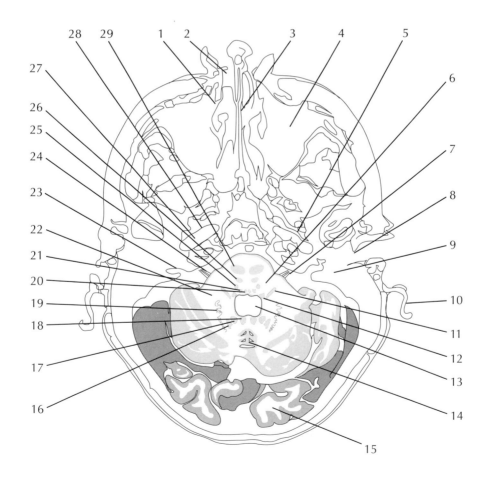

of motor and sensory (intermediate) parts.[1] (pp. 416–419), 4 (p. 1070)

25. *Facial nucleus.* Contains motor neurons that innervate the muscles of facial expression.[2] (pp. 322–330)

26. *Medial lemniscus.* Transits touch and proprioception for the contralateral side of the body.[1] (pp. 203–206)

27. *Internal carotid artery.* Supplies eye and associated tissues, pituitary gland, and anterior portion of the brain.[4] (p. 686)

28. *Carotid canal.* Provides for the internal carotid artery to enter the skull.[9] (p. 680)

29. *Pyramidal (corticospinal) tract.* Pathway for the control of contralateral voluntary motor activity for the body.[2] (pp. 208–210), 3 (p. 193), 12 (p. 148)

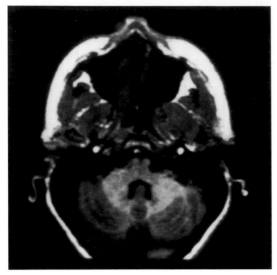

MRI

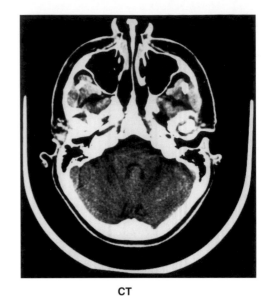

CT

25   1   2   3

24

4

5

23

6

22

7

21

20

19

8

18

9

17

10

16

11

12

15   14   13

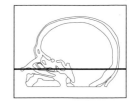

Axial 15

1. *Nasal septum.* Separates the right and left nasal fossae (cavities).[14] (p. 1402)

2. *Pons.* Contains neural circuits that transmit information between the spinal cord and higher brain regions. Regulates levels of arousal, blood pressure, and respiration.[2] (p. 9), [11] (p. 181)

3. *Middle cerebellar peduncle.* Connects cerebellum to pons, relaying input from the contralateral cerebral cortex to the lateral lobe of the cerebellum.[2] (pp. 242, 249), [11] (p. 13), [12] (pp. 104–105)

4. *Pyramidal (corticospinal) tract.* Pathway for the control of contralateral voluntary motor activity for the body.[2] (p. 208–210), [3] (p. 193), [12] (p. 148)

5. *Medial lemniscus.* Transits touch and proprioception for the contralateral side of the body.[1] (p. 203–206)

6. *Lateral lemniscus.* Transmits auditory information.[1] (p. 264), [3] (p. 199)

7. *External auditory (acoustic) meatus.* Essential for the effective mechanical responses of the tympanic membrane.[4] (p. 1192)

8. *Auricle.* Collects air vibrations.[14] (p. 167)

9. *Facial nucleus.* Contains motor neurons that innervate the muscles of facial expression.[2] (pp. 322–330)

10. *Medial longitudinal fasciculus.* Brainstem pathway essential for the control of eye movements.[2] (p. 173)

11. *Choroid plexus of the fourth ventricle.* Produces cerebrospinal fluid (CSF).[5] (p. 102), [14] (p. 1213)

12. *Fourth ventricle.* Cavity filled with CSF.[7] (p. 70), [13] (p. 97)

13. *Cerebellar vermis.* Regulates and coordinates axial and girdle musculature.[3] (p. 282), [7] (p. 290)

14. *Occipital lobe.* Involved in the higher order processing of visual information.[6] (pp. 21–22)

15. *Cerebellar hemisphere.* Involved with movements of the extremities and fine coordinated movements.[3] (p. 283), [12] (p. 175), [15] (p. 633–634)

16. *Auditory nucleus (VIII) (vestibular).* Transmits information involved with equilibrium.[3] (p. 199)

17. *Auditory nucleus (VIII) (cochlear).* Important in localizing and recognizing patterns of sound.[2] (pp. 166–167), [3] (p. 199)

18. *Inferior cerebellar peduncle.* Connects the cerebellum to the medulla, and is important in maintaining equilibrium.[2] (pp. 242, 249), [11] (p. 13), [12] (pp. 104–105), [20] (pp. 326–327)

19. *Vestibule.* Important in maintaining balance and equilibrium.[9] (pp. 775–776)

20. *Semicircular canal.* Concerned with the maintenance of balance.[6] (pp. 210–217), [9] (pp. 774–776)

21. *Cochlea (acoustic labyrinth).* The primary organ of hearing.[1] (p. 254), [8] (pp. 374–375, 379), [14] (p. 334)

22. *Pontine cistern.* CSF-filled space located between the pons and the upper clivus.[10] (pp. 115–116)

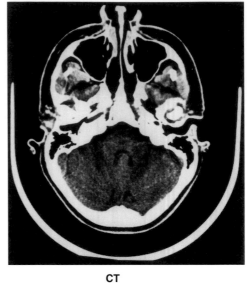

MRI

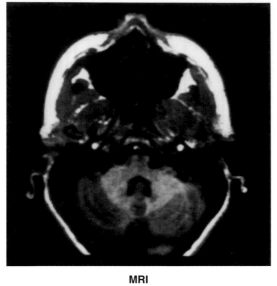

CT

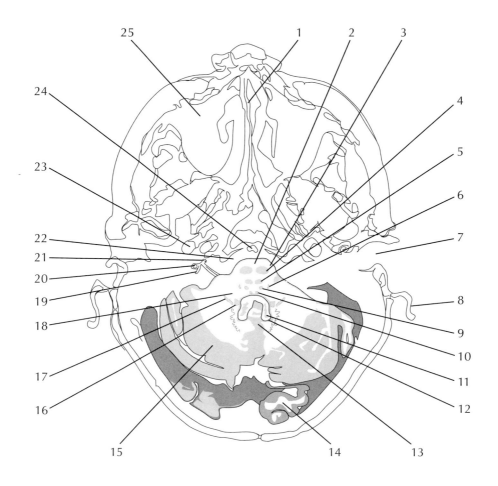

25   1   2   3

24

23

22

21

20

19

18

17

16

15   14   13

4

5

6

7

8

9

10

11

12

23. *Internal carotid artery.* Supplies eye and associated tissues, pituitary gland, and anterior portion of the brain.[4] [(p. 686)]

24. *Basilar artery.* Blood supply to upper medulla, pons, cerebellum, inner ear, occipital lobe, and part of temporal lobe.[5] [(p. 1042)]

25. *Maxillary sinus.* Acts as a resonator to the voice.[23] [(pp. 734–736)]

.

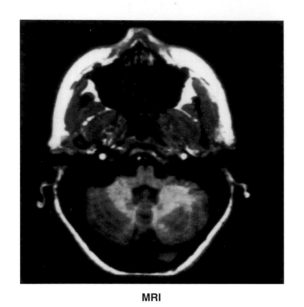

MRI

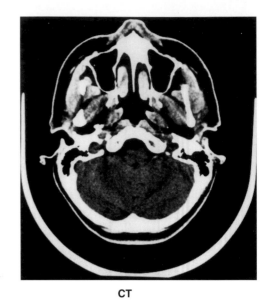

CT

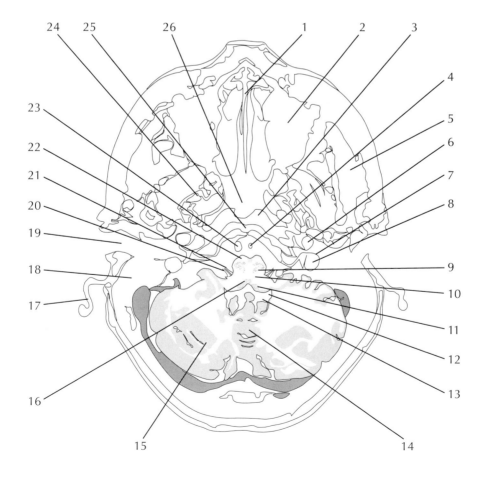

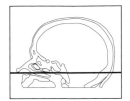

Axial 16

1. *Nasal septum.* Separates the right and left nasal fossae (cavities).[14 (p. 1402)]

2. *Maxillary sinus.* Acts as a resonator to the voice.[23 (pp. 734–736)]

3. *Longus capitis muscle.* Serves to flex the head.[4 (p. 541), 8 (p. 211)]

4. *Vertebral artery.* Provides branches to the head and neck, including spinal and muscular arteries.[4 (pp. 694–696), 10 (pp. 228–229)]

5. *Masseter muscle.* Used in biting and chewing.[14 (p. 534)]

6. *Internal carotid artery.* Supplies eye and associated tissues, pituitary gland, and anterior portion of the brain.[4 (p. 686)]

7. *Jugular foramen.* Transmits the inferior petrosal sinus, the glossopharyngeal, vagus, and accessory nerves, and the internal jugular vein.[4 (pp. 307, 312, 329)]

8. *Internal jugular vein.* The primary venous drainage of the brain, face, and neck.[4 (p. 741), 8 (pp. 435, 438)]

9. *Inferior olivary nucleus.* Involved in adaptive motor behavior.[1 (pp. 363–366), 6 (pp. 349–350)]

10. *Reticular formation.* Involved in sleep and arousal activities, the motor system, and regulation of visceral activities.[2 (p. 229), 12 (p. 148)]

11. *Hypoglossal nucleus.* Innervates the intrinsic muscles of the tongue.[2 (pp. 322–333)]

12. *Foramina of Luschka (foramina of Key and Retzius).* Outlets of the ventricular system to the subarachnoid space.[1 (p. 174), 14 (p. 117)]

13. *Fourth ventricle.* Cavity filled with cerebrospinal fluid.[7 (p. 70), 13 (p. 97)]

14. *Cerebellar vermis.* Regulates and coordinates axial and girdle musculature.[3 (p. 282), 7 (p. 290)]

15. *Cerebellar hemisphere.* Involved with movements of the extremities and fine coordinated movements.[3 (p. 283), 12 (p. 175), 15 (pp. 633–634)]

16. *Medial longitudinal fasciculus.* Brainstem pathway essential for the control of eye movements.[2 (p. 173)]

17. *Auricle.* Collects air vibrations.[14 (p. 167)]

18. *Mastoid process.* Contains air cells (sinuses) and serves as the attachment for the sternocleidomastoid, splenius capitis, and longus capitis muscles.[4 (pp. 307, 328), 8 (p. 121)]

19. *External auditory (acoustic) meatus.* Essential for the effective mechanical responses of the tympanic membrane.[4 (p. 1192)]

20. *Vagus nerve (cranial nerve X).* Provides innervation to the thorax and abdomen, the pharynx and larynx, external ear, and taste buds on the epiglottis.[1 (p. 423), 4 (pp. 1076–1080)]

21. *Glossopharyngeal nerve (cranial nerve IX).* Innervates portions of the tongue and pharynx.[1 (p. 420), 20 (pp. 244–246)]

22. *Pyramidal (corticospinal) tract.* Pathway for the control of contralateral voluntary motor activity for the body.[2 (pp. 208–210), 3 (p. 193), 12 (p. 148)]

23. *Basilar artery.* Blood supply to upper

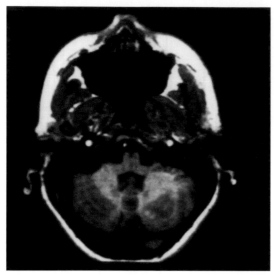

MRI

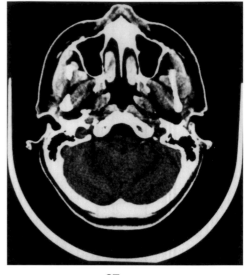

CT

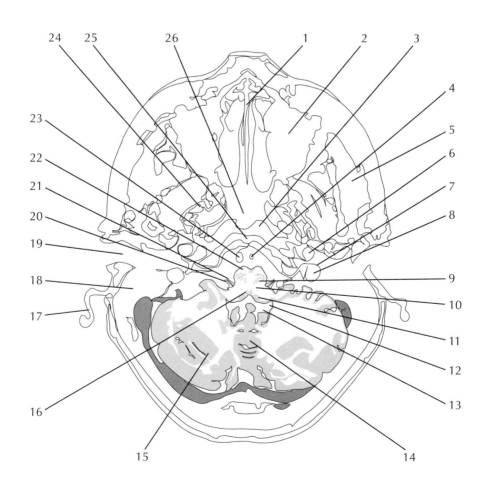

medulla, pons, cerebellum, inner ear, occipital lobe, and part of temporal lobe.[15] (p. 1042)

24. *Pterygopalatine fossa.* Contains the pterygopalatine ganglion, the terminal branches of the maxillary artery, and the second division of the trigeminal nerve.[9] (p. 752)

25. *Clivus of sphenoid bone.* Supports the medulla oblongata and the lower pons.[4] (p. 320), [14] (p. 328)

26. *Nasopharynx.* Assists in respiration.[8] (pp. 468–469), [24] (p. 462)

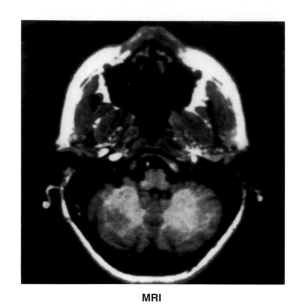

MRI

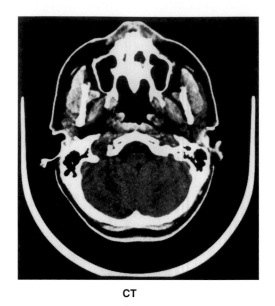

CT

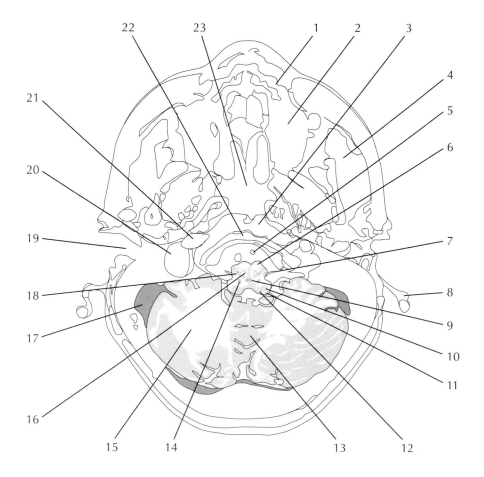

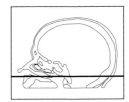

Axial 17

1. *Alveolar process of the maxilla.* Origin of the buccinator muscle.[4 (pp. 338–340)]

2. *Maxillary sinus.* Acts as a resonator to the voice.[23 (pp. 734–736)]

3. *Longus capitis muscle.* Serves to flex the head.[4 (p. 541), 8 (p. 211)]

4. *Masseter muscle.* Used in biting and chewing.[4 (p. 534)]

5. *Vertebral artery.* Provides branches to the head and neck, including spinal and muscular arteries.[4 (pp. 694–696), 10 (pp. 228–229)]

6. *Pyramidal (corticospinal) tract.* Pathway for the control of contralateral voluntary motor activity for the body.[2 (pp. 208–210), 3 (p. 193), 12 (p. 148)]

7. *Hypoglossal nerve (cranial nerve XII).* The motor nerve of the tongue providing innervation of the musculature.[14 (p. 1083), 24 (p. 429)]

8. *Auricle.* Collects air vibrations.[14 (p. 167)]

9. *Medial lemniscus.* Transmits touch and proprioception for the contralateral side of the body.[1 (pp. 203–206)]

10. *Cuneate nucleus.* Major relay for touch discrimination and proprioception from the upper extremities.[2 (pp. 121–122), 3 (p. 203)]

11. *Cuneate fasciculus.* Transmits touch discrimination and proprioception from the upper extremities.[2 (pp. 121–122), 3 (p. 203)]

12. *Gracile nucleus.* Major relay for touch discrimination, and proprioception from the lower extremities.[2 (pp. 121–122), 3 (p. 203)]

13. *Cerebellar vermis.* Regulates and coordinates axial and girdle musculature.[3 (p. 282), 7 (p. 290)]

14. *Nucleus ambiguus.* Provides for innervation of muscles of the palate, pharynx, and larynx.[2 (pp. 222–333)]

15. *Cerebellar hemisphere.* Involved with movements of the extremities and fine coordinated movements.[3 (p. 283), 12 (p. 175), 15 (pp. 633–634)]

16. *Accessory olivary nucleus.* Assists in motor coordination.[3 (p. 203)]

17. *Sigmoid venous sinus.* Receives most of the blood supply from the dural venous sinuses.[1 (pp. 187–188), 17 (p. 867)]

18. *Inferior olivary nucleus.* Involved in adaptive motor behavior.[1 (pp. 363–366), 6 (pp. 349–350)]

19. *External auditory (acoustic) meatus.* Essential for the effective mechanical responses of the tympanic membrane.[4 (p. 1192)]

20. *Jugular foramen.* Transmits the inferior petrosal sinus, the glossopharyngeal, vagus, and accessory nerves, and the internal jugular vein.[4 (pp. 307, 312, 329)]

21. *Internal carotid artery.* Supplies eye and associated tissues, pituitary gland, and anterior portion of the brain.[4 (p. 686)]

22. *Clivus of the sphenoid bone.* Supports the medulla oblongata and the lower pons.[4 (p. 320), 14 (p. 328)]

23. *Nasopharynx.* Assists in respiration.[8 (p. 468), 24 (p. 462)]

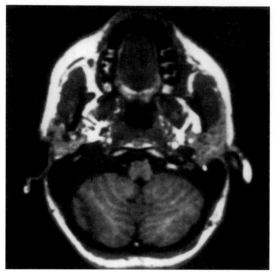

MRI

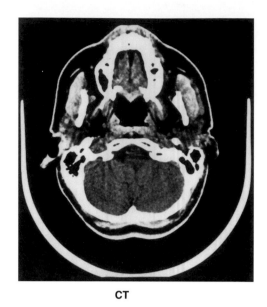

CT

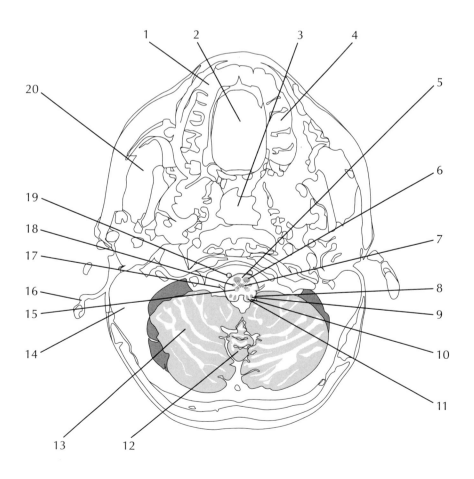

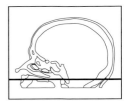

Axial 18

1. *Alveolar process of the maxilla.* Origin of the buccinator muscle.[4 (pp. 338–340)]

2. *Hard palate.* Together with the soft palate forms the roof of the mouth.[4 (p. 1270), 8 (p. 467)]

3. *Nasopharynx.* Assists in respiration.[8 (pp. 468–469), 24 (p. 462)]

4. *Teeth.* Represent the organs of mastication and are influential in articulation of speech.[8 (pp. 460–461)]

5. *Reticular formation.* Involved in sleep and arousal activities, the motor system, and regulation of visceral activities.[2 (p. 229), 12 (p. 148)]

6. *Pyramidal (corticospinal) tract.* Pathway for the control of contralateral voluntary motor activity for the body.[2 (pp. 208–210), 3 (p. 193), 12 (p. 148)]

7. *Pyramidal decussation.* Allows one side of the brain to control the opposite side of the body.[12 (p. 336)]

8. *Cuneate fasciculus.* Transmits touch discrimination and proprioception from the upper extremities.[2 (pp. 121–122), 3 (p. 203)]

9. *Cuneate nucleus.* Major relay for touch discrimination and proprioception from the upper extremities.[2 (pp. 121–122), 3 (p. 203)]

10. *Gracile fasciculus.* Transmits touch discrimination and proprioception from the lower extremities.[2 (pp. 121–122), 3 (p. 203)]

11. *Gracile nucleus.* Major relay for touch discrimination and proprioception from the lower extremities.[2 (pp. 121–122), 3 (p. 203)]

12. *Cerebellar vermis.* Regulates and coordinates axial and girdle musculature.[3 (p. 282), 7 (p. 290)]

13. *Cerebellar hemisphere.* Involved with movements of the extremities and fine coordinated movements.[3 (p. 283), 12 (p. 175), 15 (pp. 633–634)]

14. *Mastoid process.* Contains air cells (sinuses) and serves as the attachment for the sternocleidomastoid, splenius capitis, and longus capitis muscles.[4 (pp. 307, 328), 8 (p. 121)]

15. *Pyramidal corticospinal tract (lateral corticospinal tract).* Pathway for the control of contralateral voluntary motor activity for the body.[2 (p. 208–210), 3 (p. 193), 12 (p. 148)]

16. *Auricle.* Collects air vibrations.[14 (p. 167)]

17. *Accessory nerve (spinal accessory nerve, cranial nerve XI).* Fibers from the motor neurons of the accessory nucleus and the nucleus ambiguus.[2 (pp. 322–330)]

18. *Accessory nucleus.* Motor neurons of the accessory nerve.[2 (pp. 322–330)]

19. *Vertebral artery.* Provides branches to the head and neck, including spinal and muscular arteries.[4 (pp. 694–696), 10 (pp. 228–229)]

20. *Masseter muscle.* Used in biting and chewing.[4 (p. 534)]

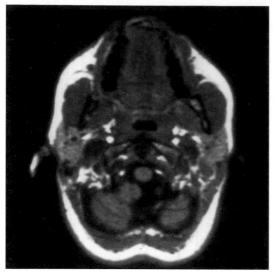

MRI

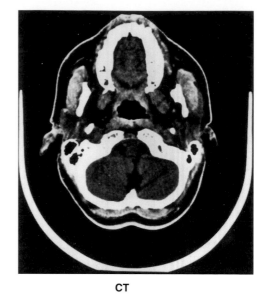

CT

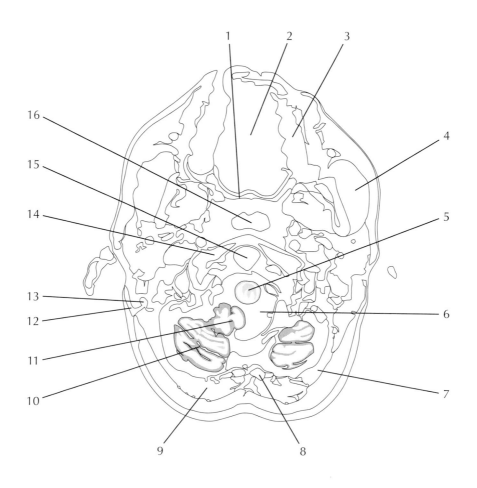

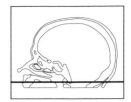

Axial 19

1. *Soft palate.* Plays an important role in swallowing, speech, blowing air out through the mouth while preventing release through the nose.[4] (pp. 1270, 1313), [8] (p. 467)

2. *Hard palate.* Together with the soft palate forms the roof of the mouth.[4] (p. 1270), [8] (p. 467)

3. *Maxilla.* Forms the upper jaw, most of the roof of the mouth, the floor and the lateral walls of the nasal cavity, and the floor of the orbit.[4] (pp. 338–340)

4. *Masseter muscle.* Used in biting and chewing.[4] (p. 534)

5. *Spinal cord.* Innervates the motor and sensory areas of the body.[1] (p. 117), [4] (p. 864)

6. *Foramen magnum.* Connects the cranial cavity with the spinal canal.[9] (pp. 680–681)

7. *Rectus capitis posterior major muscle.* Serves to extend and rotate the head.[4] (pp. 546–547), [8] (pp. 211, 255–268)

8. *Rectus capitis posterior minor muscle.* Serves to extend the head.[4] (pp. 546–547), [8] (pp. 211, 255–268)

9. *Semispinalis capitis muscle.* Serves to extend and rotate the head.[4] (p. 545), [8] (pp. 211, 255–268)

10. *Cerebellar hemisphere.* Involved with movements of the extremities and fine coordinated movements.[3] (p. 283), [12] (p. 175), [15] (pp. 633–634)

11. *Cerebellar tonsil.* Concerned with guiding limb movement and posture.[2] (p. 242)

12. *Sternocleidomastoid muscle.* Unilateral action of the muscle draws the head to the side, while bilateral contraction serves to flex the vertebral column, the head, and elevate the chin.[4] (pp. 538–539), [8] (pp. 208, 255–268)

13. *Digastric muscle (posterior belly).* Raises the hyoid bone and depresses the mandible.[8] (pp. 121–123), [17] (p. 815)

14. *Atlas (C1).* Provides support for the head.[4] (pp. 273–274), [8] (pp. 129–130)

15. *Odontoid process (dens) of axis (C2).* Serves as the pivot around which the atlas rotates.[4] (pp. 273–274), [8] (pp. 129–130)

16. *Oropharynx.* Receives food from the mouth and air from the nasopharynx.[4] (p. 1309), [8] (pp. 468–469)

Coronal Views

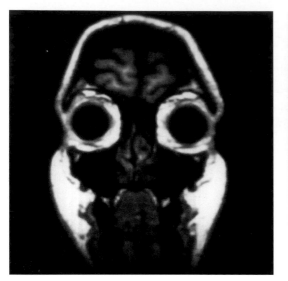

MRI

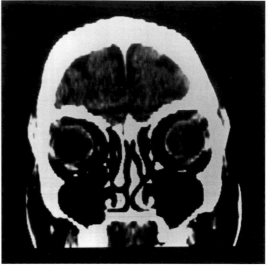

CT

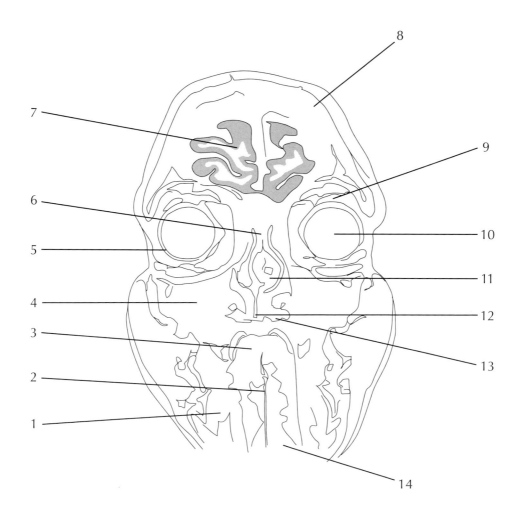

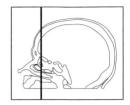

Coronal 1

1. *Mandible.* Serves as an attachment for muscles of mastication.[8] (p. 123), [17] (p. 815)

2. *Septum of the tongue.* Divides the tongue in half.[9] (p. 746), [14] (p. 1402)

3. *Genioglossus muscle.* Serves to retract, depress, and protrude the tongue as well as to elevate the hyoid bone.[4] (p. 1304), [8] (pp. 204–205, 257)

4. *Maxillary sinus.* Acts as a resonator to the voice.[23] (pp. 734–736)

5. *Globe.* Complex structure for vision.[8] (pp. 380–384), [25] (p. 188)

6. *Superior nasal concha.* Forms the upper boundary of the superior meatus.[14] (p. 348), [17] (p. 952)

7. *Frontal lobe.* Involved in personality, insight, and foresight; initiation of voluntary movements; written and spoken language.[6] (pp. 18–20)

8. *Frontal bone.* Provides enclosure and protection of the brain.[24] (p. 170)

9. *Superior muscle bundle.* Contains superior rectus (superior and medial orbit deviation), and superior oblique muscles (inferior and lateral orbit deviation).[25] (p. 189)   .

10. *Vitreous body (eye).* Forms most of the eyeball, transmits light, holds the retina in place, and provides support for the lens.[9] (p. 714)

11. *Middle nasal concha.* Separates the superior and middle nasal meatus.[14] (p. 348), [17] (p. 952)

12. *Nasal septum.* Separates the right and left nasal fossae (cavities).[14] (p. 1402)

13. *Inferior nasal concha.* Forms the lower part of the lateral wall of the nasal cavity.[4] (p. 348), [17] (p. 952)

14. *Anterior belly of the digastric muscle.* Raises the hyoid bone and depresses the mandible.[9] (pp. 665–667)

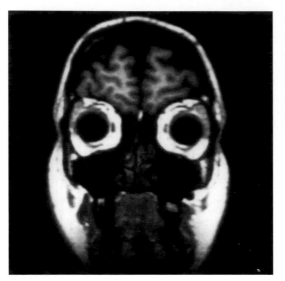

MRI

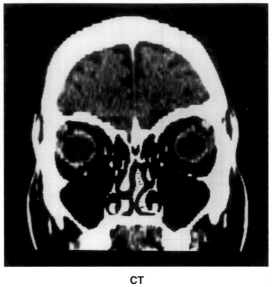

CT

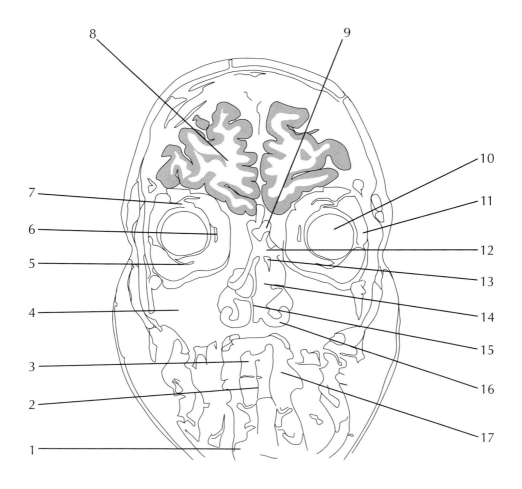

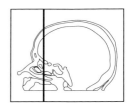

Coronal 2

1. *Anterior belly of the digastric muscle.* Raises the hyoid bone and depresses the mandible.[9] (pp. 665–667)

2. *Septum of the tongue.* Divides the tongue in half.[9] (p. 746), [14] (p. 1402)

3. *Body of the tongue.* Involved in taste, speaking, swallowing, chewing, and oral cleansing.[9] (p. 745)

4. *Maxillary sinus.* Acts as a resonator to the voice.[23] (pp. 734–736)

5. *Inferior oblique muscle.* Serves to elevate the medially rotated eye and to abduct and rotate the eye laterally.[9] (pp. 715–717)

6. *Medial rectus muscle.* Rotates the eye so that the cornea is directed medially.[9] (p. 715), [25] (p. 189)

7. *Superior muscle bundle.* Contains superior rectus (superior and medial orbit deviation) and superior oblique muscles (inferior and lateral orbit deviation).[25] (p. 189)

8. *Frontal lobe.* Involved in personality, insight, and foresight; initiation of voluntary movements; written and spoken language.[6] (pp. 18–20)

9. *Superior nasal meatus.* Serves to warm and moisturize inspired air.[4] (pp. 313–314), [14] (p. 920)

10. *Globe.* Complex structure for vision.[8] (pp. 380–384), [25] (p. 188)

11. *Lateral rectus.* Rotates the eye so that the cornea is directed laterally.[9] (p. 715), [25] (p. 189)

12. *Superior nasal concha.* Forms the upper boundary of the superior meatus.[14] (p. 348), [17] (p. 952)

13. *Middle nasal meatus.* Aids in warming and moistening inspired air.[4] (pp. 313–314), [14] (p. 920)

14. *Middle nasal concha.* Separates the superior and middle nasal meatus.[14] (p. 348), [17] (p. 952)

15. *Inferior nasal meatus.* Aids in warming and moistening inspired air.[4] (pp. 313–314), [14] (p. 920)

16. *Inferior nasal concha.* Forms the lower part of the lateral wall of the nasal cavity.[14] (p. 348), [17] (p. 952)

17. *Genioglossus muscle.* Serves to retract, depress, and protrude the tongue as well as to elevate the hyoid bone.[4] (p. 1304), [8] (pp. 204–205, 257)

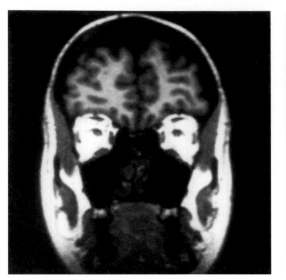

MRI

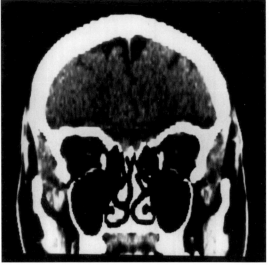

CT

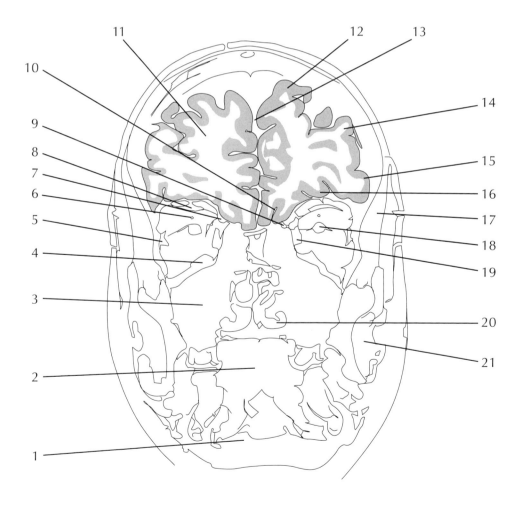

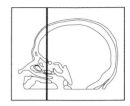

Coronal 3

1. *Anterior belly of the digastric muscle.* Raises the hyoid bone and depresses the mandible.[9] (pp. 665–667)

2. *Body of the tongue.* Involved in taste, speaking, swallowing, chewing, and oral cleansing.[9] (p. 745)

3. *Maxillary sinus.* Acts as a resonator to the voice.[23] (pp. 734–736)

4. *Inferior rectus muscle.* Serves to depress, adduct, and laterally rotate the eye.[9] (pp. 715–717)

5. *Lateral rectus muscle.* Rotates the eye so that the cornea is directed laterally.[9] (p. 715), [25] (p. 189)

6. *Superior ophthalmic vein.* Anastomoses with the facial vein and allows blood to flow in either direction because it has no valves.[9] (p. 719)

7. *Superior oblique muscle.* Depresses the medially rotated eye, rotates medially and abducts the eyeball.[9] (pp. 715–717)

8. *Superior muscle bundle.* Contains superior rectus (superior and medial orbit deviation) and superior oblique muscles (inferior and lateral orbit deviation).[25] (p. 189)

9. *Olfactory bulb.* Receives projections of the olfactory nerves.[1] (p. 293)

10. *Olfactory sulcus.* Forms the lateral margin of the gyrus rectus.[1] (p. 160)

11. *Frontal lobe.* Involved in personality, insight, and foresight; initiation of voluntary movements; written and spoken language.[6] (pp. 18–20)

12. *Superior frontal gyrus.* Participates in the control and initiation of voluntary movements and is involved in personality, insight, and judgment.[6] (pp. 18–20), [18] (p. 674), [19] (p. 260)

13. *Interhemispheric (longitudinal) fissure.* Separates the cerebral hemispheres.[12] (p. 218), [19] (p. 257)

14. *Middle frontal gyrus.* Participates in the control and initiation of voluntary movements; involved in personality, insight, and foresight.[6] (p. 18)

15. *Inferior frontal gyrus.* Important for the production of written and spoken language.[6] (p. 18)

16. *Orbital gyrus.* Involved in the conscious perception of odors.[1] (pp. 160, 296, 463)

17. *Temporalis muscle.* Assists in jaw closure.[8] (pp. 255–268)

18. *Optic nerve.* Nerve of sight.[7] (pp. 221–227)

19. *Medial rectus muscle.* Rotates the eye so that the cornea is directed medially.[9] (p. 715), [25] (p. 189)

20. *Inferior nasal concha.* Forms the lower part of the lateral wall of the nasal cavity.[14] (p. 348), [17] (p. 952)

21. *Masseter muscle.* Used in biting and chewing.[4] (p. 534)

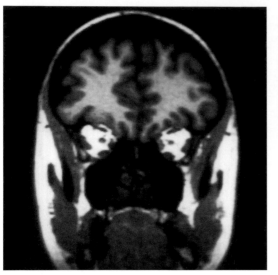

MRI

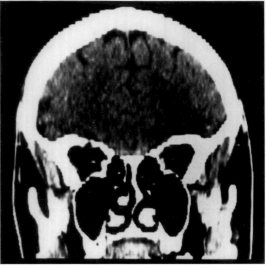

CT

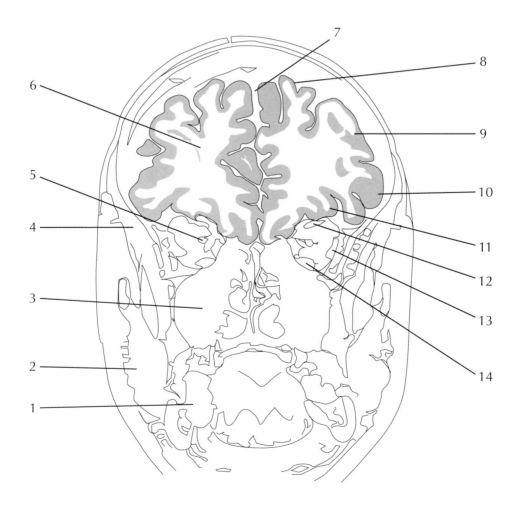

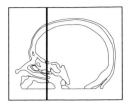

Coronal 4

1. *Mandible.* Serves as an attachment for muscles of mastication.[8] (p. 123), [17] (p. 815)

2. *Masseter muscle.* Used in biting and chewing.[4] (p. 534)

3. *Maxillary sinus.* Acts as a resonator to the voice.[23] (pp. 734–736)

4. *Temporalis muscle.* Assists in jaw closure.[8] (pp. 255–268)

5. *Optic nerve (cranial nerve II).* Nerve of sight.[7] (pp. 221, 227)

6. *Frontal lobe.* Involved in personality, insight, and foresight; initiation of voluntary movements; written and spoken language.[6] (pp. 18–20)

7. *Interhemispheric (longitudinal) fissure.* Separates the cerebral hemispheres.[12] (p. 218), [19] (p. 257)

8. *Superior frontal gyrus.* Participates in the control and initiation of voluntary movements and is involved in personality, insight, and judgment.[6] (pp. 18–20), [18] (p. 674), [19] (p. 260)

9. *Middle frontal gyrus.* Participates in the control and initiation of voluntary movements; involved in personality, insight, and foresight.[6] (p. 18)

10. *Inferior frontal gyrus.* Important for the production of written and spoken language.[6] (p. 18)

11. *Orbital gyrus.* Involved in the conscious perception of odors.[1] (pp. 160, 296, 493)

12. *Superior muscle bundle.* Contains superior rectus (superior and medial orbit deviation) and superior oblique muscles (inferior and lateral orbit deviation).[25] (p. 189)

13. *Lateral rectus muscle.* Rotates the eye so that the cornea is directed laterally.[9] (p. 715), [25] (p. 189)

14. *Inferior rectus muscle.* Serves to depress, adduct, and laterally rotate the eye.[9] (pp. 715–717)

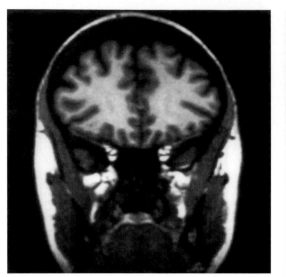
MRI

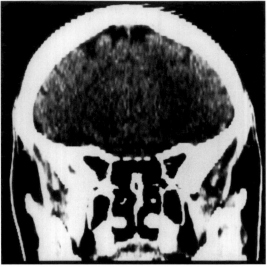
CT

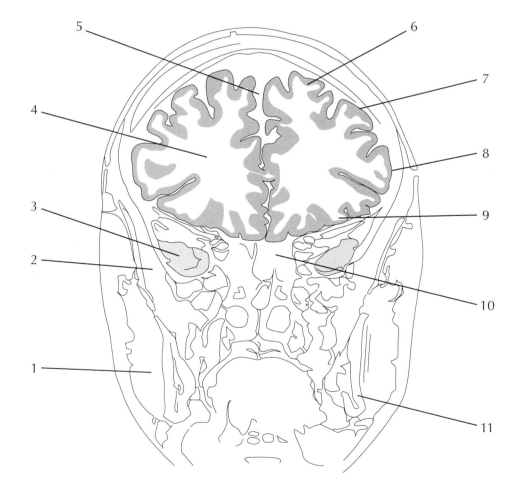

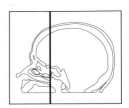

Coronal 5

1. *Masseter muscle.* Used in biting and chewing.[4] (p. 534)

2. *Temporalis muscle.* Assists in jaw closure.[8] (pp. 255–268)

3. *Temporal lobe.* Involved in emotions, visceral responses, learning, and memory.[6] (pp. 21–22)

4. *Frontal lobe.* Involved in personality, insight, and foresight; initiation of voluntary movements; written and spoken language.[6] (pp. 18–20)

5. *Interhemispheric (longitudinal) fissure.* Separates the cerebral hemispheres.[12] (p. 218), [19] (p. 257)

6. *Superior frontal gyrus.* Participates in the control and initiation of voluntary movements and is involved in personality, insight, and judgment.[6] (pp. 18–20), [18] (p. 674), [19] (p. 260)

7. *Middle frontal gyrus.* Participates in the control and initiation of voluntary movements; involved in personality, insight, and foresight.[6] (p. 18)

8. *Inferior frontal gyrus.* Important for the production of written and spoken language.[6] (p. 18)

9. *Orbital gyrus.* Involved in the conscious perception of odors.[1] (pp. 160, 296, 493)

10. *Sphenoid sinus.* Acts as a resonator to the voice.[23] (pp. 734–736)

11. *Angle of the mandible.* Insertion of the masseter and medial pterygoid muscles.[4] (p. 316)

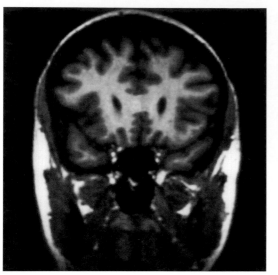

MRI

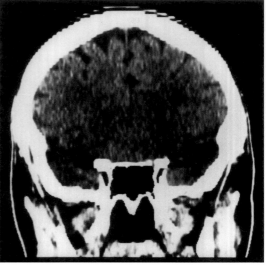

CT

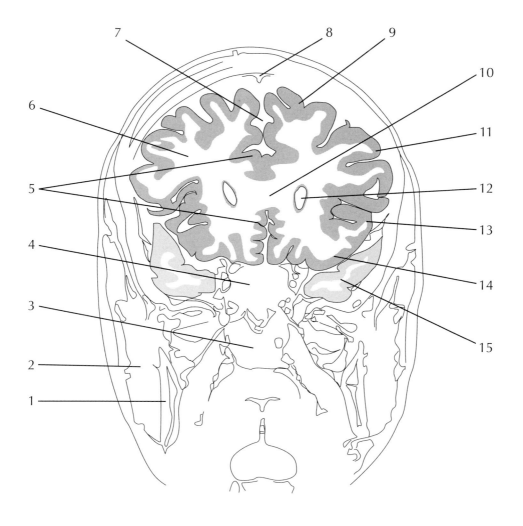

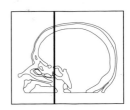

Coronal 6

1. *Mandible.* Serves as an attachment for muscles of mastication.[8] (p. 123), [17] (p. 815)

2. *Masseter muscle.* Used in biting and chewing.[4] (p. 534)

3. *Nasopharynx.* Assists in respiration.[8] (pp. 468–469), [24] (p. 462)

4. *Sphenoid sinus.* Acts as a resonator to the voice.[23] (pp. 734–736)

5. *Cingulate gyrus.* Plays a role in emotional behavior, the autonomic nervous system, learning, and memory.[12] (p. 272), [18] (pp. 255, 674)

6. *Frontal lobe.* Involved in personality, insight, and foresight; initiation of voluntary movements; written and spoken language.[6] (pp. 18–20)

7. *Interhemispheric (longitudinal) fissure.* Separates the cerebral hemispheres.[12] (p. 218), [19] (p. 257)

8. *Superior sagittal sinus.* Drains blood from the brain and drains cerebrospinal fluid from the subarachnoid space.[11] (pp. 292, 439)

9. *Superior frontal gyrus.* Participates in the control and initiation of voluntary movements and is involved in personality, insight, and judgment.[6] (pp. 18–20), [18] (p. 674), [19] (p. 260)

10. *Genu of the corpus callosum.* Connects the frontal lobes.[2] (pp. 51, 131), [12] (p. 248), [15] (p. 365), [19] (p. 269)

11. *Middle frontal gyrus.* Participates in the control and initiation of voluntary movements; involved in personality, insight, and foresight.[6] (p. 18)

12. *Anterior horn of the lateral ventricle.* Anterior ependymal-lined cavity.[1] (pp. 172–173), [11] (p. 283), [12] (pp. 253–256)

13. *Inferior frontal gyrus.* Important for the production of written and spoken language.[6] (p. 18)

14. *Orbital gyrus.* Involved in the conscious perception of odors.[1] (pp. 160, 296, 493)

15. *Temporal lobe.* Involved in emotions, visceral responses, learning, and memory.[6] (pp. 21–22)

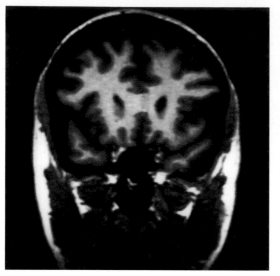

MRI

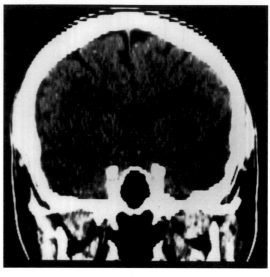

CT

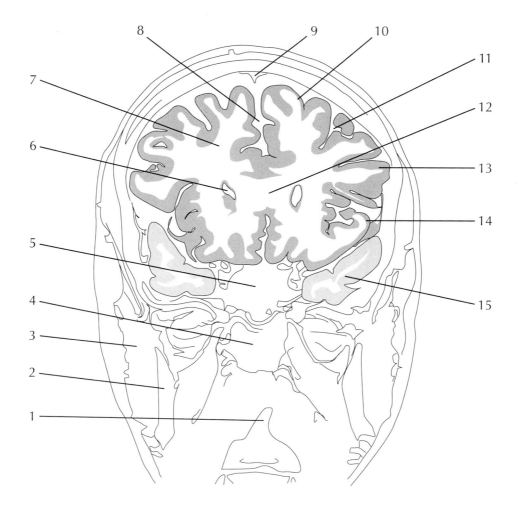

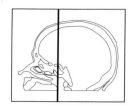

Coronal 7

1. *Oropharynx.* Receives food from the mouth and air from the nasopharynx.[4 (p. 1309), 8 (pp. 468–469)]

2. *Mandible.* Serves as an attachment for muscles of mastication.[8 (p. 123), 17 (p. 815)]

3. *Masseter muscle.* Used in biting and chewing.[4 (p. 534)]

4. *Nasopharynx.* Assists in respiration.[8 (pp. 468–469), 24 (p. 462)]

5. *Sphenoid sinus.* Acts as a resonator to the voice.[23 (pp. 734–736)]

6. *Anterior horn of the lateral ventricle.* Anterior ependymal-lined cavity.[1 (pp. 172–173), 11 (p. 283), 12 (pp. 253–256)]

7. *Frontal lobe.* Involved in personality, insight, and foresight; initiation of voluntary movements; written and spoken language.[6 (pp. 18–20)]

8. *Interhemispheric (longitudinal) fissure.* Separates the cerebral hemispheres.[12 (p. 218), 19 (p. 257)]

9. *Superior sagittal sinus.* Drains blood from the brain and drains cerebrospinal fluid from the subarachnoid space.[11 (pp. 292, 439)]

10. *Superior frontal gyrus.* Participates in the control and initiation of voluntary movements and is involved in personality, insight, and judgment.[6 (18–20), 18 (p. 674), 19 (p. 260)]

11. *Superior frontal sulcus.* Separates the superior frontal gyrus from the middle frontal gyrus.[12 (p. 219)]

12. *Genu of the corpus callosum.* Connects the frontal lobes.[2 (pp. 51, 131), 12 (p. 248), 15 (p. 365), 19 (p. 269)]

13. *Middle frontal gyrus.* Participates in the control and initiation of voluntary movements; involved in personality, insight, and foresight.[6 (p. 18)]

14. *Inferior frontal gyrus.* Important for the production of written and spoken language.[6 (p. 18)]

15. *Temporal lobe.* Involved in emotions, visceral responses, learning, and memory.[6 (pp. 21–22)]

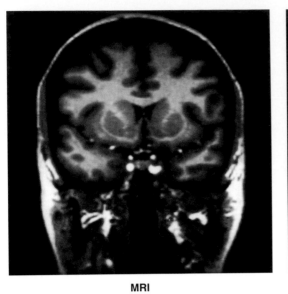
MRI

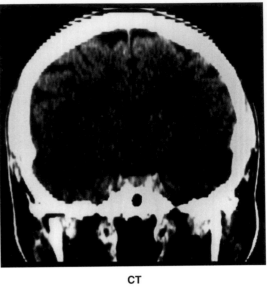
CT

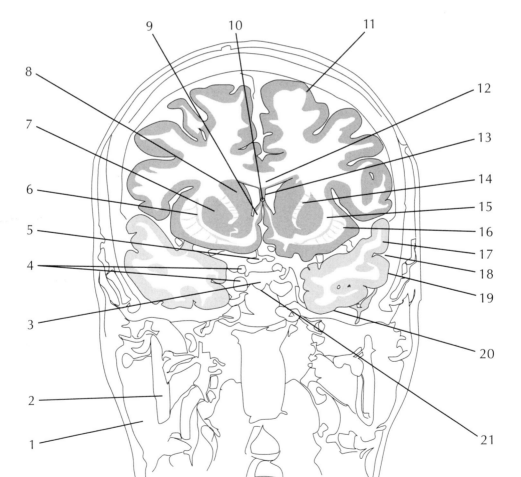

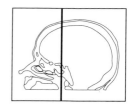

Coronal 8

1. *Masseter muscle.* Used in biting and chewing.[4] (p. 534)

2. *Mandible.* Serves as an attachment for muscles of mastication.[7] (p. 815), [16] (p. 123)

3. *Pituitary gland (hypophysis).* Consists of an anterior lobe (adenohypophysis), a nonfunctional pars intermedia, and the posterior lobe (neurohypophysis).[1] (pp. 421–424), [2] (p. 350), [12] (pp. 201–203)

4. *Internal carotid artery.* Supplies the eye and associated tissues, pituitary gland, and anterior portion of the brain.[4] (p. 686)

5. *Optic chiasm.* Convergence of the optic nerves.[2] (p. 143), [11] (p. 227)

6. *Claustrum.* Involved in mediating visual attention.[11] (p. 244), [15] (p. 460)

7. *Putamen.* Involved in motor function.[6] (p. 304), [7] (p. 11)

8. *Caudate nucleus.* Involved in cognitive functions and movement.[6] (p. 304), [7] (p. 11), [12] (pp. 207–212), [15] (pp. 306–307), [18] (pp. 523–524)

9. *Fornix.* Efferent tract of the hippocampus projecting to the mamillary bodies.[11] (p. 276), [12] (pp. 268–269), [19] (p. 269)

10. *Anterior commissure.* A neocortical "corpus callosum."[11] (p. 246), [12] (pp. 249–250)

11. *Superior frontal gyrus.* Participates in the control and initiation of voluntary movements and is involved in personality, insight, and judgment.[6] (pp. 17–20), [18] (p. 674), [19] (p. 260)

12. *Body of the corpus callosum.* Interconnects the cerebral hemispheres.[2] (pp. 51, 131), [3] (p. 248), [16] (p. 33)

13. *Septal nuclei.* A possible location for the "pleasure center" and may be involved in feeding or reproductive behavior.[1] (pp. 493–494), [2] (pp. 385–386)

14. *Internal capsule—anterior limb.* Connects subcortical nuclei with the cerebral cortex and the cerebral cortex with subcortical structures.[7] (p. 12), [11] (p. 249), [16] (p. 538)

15. *External capsule.* Consists of mainly association fibers, projection fibers, and commissural fibers.[2] (p. 276), [12] (p. 209), [13] (p. 79)

16. *Extreme capsule.* Contains corticocortical association fibers.[2] (p. 276), [12] (p. 209)

17. *Superior temporal gyrus.* The primary auditory cortex.[1] (p. 161)

18. *Superior temporal sulcus.* Serves to separate the superior and middle temporal gyri.[1] (p. 161)

19 *Middle temporal gyrus.* Functions as one of the multimodal association areas.[22] (p. 107)

20. *Inferior temporal gyrus.* Involved in the analysis of the form and color of visual stimuli.[2] (pp. 154–157), [12] (p. 219)

21. *Pituitary fossa.* Contains the pituitary gland.[9] (p. 676)

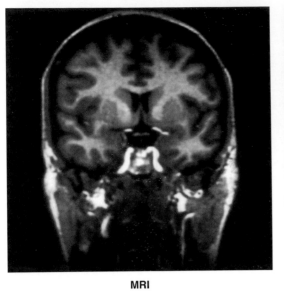

MRI

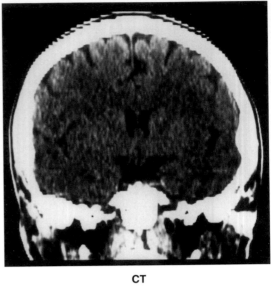

CT

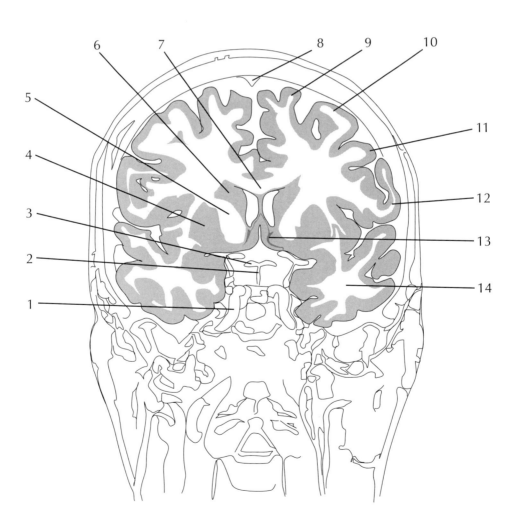

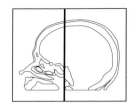

Coronal 9

1. *Internal carotid artery.* Supplies the eye and associated tissues, pituitary gland, and anterior portion of the brain.[4] (p. 686)

2. *Infundibulum (pituitary stalk, hypophyseal stalk).* Connects the pituitary gland to the hypothalamus.[2] (p. 355), [12] (p. 196), [15] (p. 739)

3. *Optic chiasm.* Convergence of the optic nerves.[2] (p. 143), [11] (p. 227)

4. *Putamen.* Involved in motor function.[6] (p. 304), [7] (p. 11)

5. *Internal capsule—genu.* Contains cortico-bulbar and corticoreticular connection fibers.[7] (p. 12), [11] (p. 249), [16] (p. 538)

6. *Caudate nucleus.* Involved in cognitive functions and movement.[6] (p. 304), [7] (p. 11), [12] (pp. 207–212), [15] (pp. 306–307), [18] (pp. 523–524)

7. *Body of corpus callosum.* Interconnects the cerebral hemispheres.[2] (pp. 51, 131), [12] (p. 248), [16] (p. 33)

8. *Superior sagittal sinus.* Drains blood from the brain and drains cerebrospinal fluid from the subarachnoid space.[11] (pp. 292, 439)

9. *Superior frontal gyrus.* Participates in the control and initiation of voluntary movements and is involved in personality, insight, and judgment.[6] (pp. 18–20), [18] (p. 674), [19] (p. 260)

10. *Precentral gyrus.* Location of the primary motor cortex.[1] (pp. 157, 326–327)

11. *Middle frontal gyrus.* Participates in the control and initiation of voluntary movements; involved in personality, insight, and foresight.[6] (p. 18)

12. *Inferior frontal gyrus.* Important for the production of written and spoken language.[6] (p. 18)

13. *Fornix.* Efferent tract of the hippocampus projecting to the mamillary bodies.[11] (p. 276), [12] (pp. 268–269), [19] (p. 269)

14. *Temporal lobe.* Involved in emotions, visceral responses, learning, and memory.[6] (pp. 21–22)

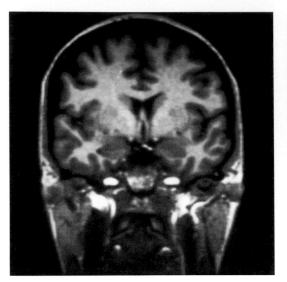

MRI

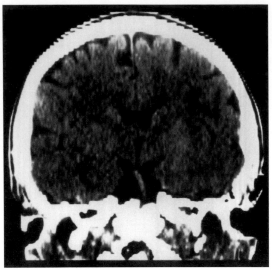

CT

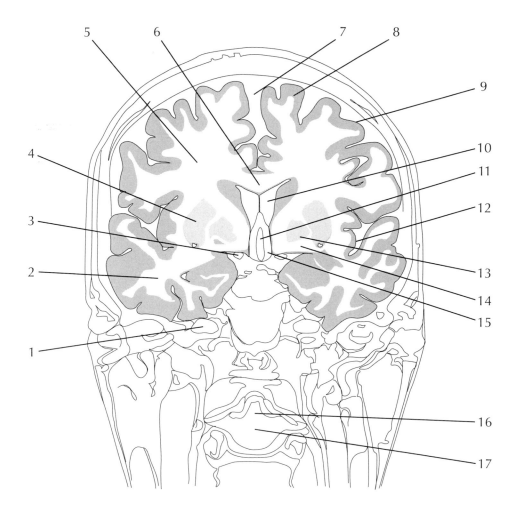

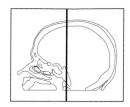

Coronal 10

1. *Internal carotid artery.* Supplies eye and associated tissues, pituitary gland, and anterior portion of the brain.[4] (p. 686)

2. *Temporal lobe.* Involved in emotions, visceral responses, learning, and memory.[6] (p. 21–22)

3. *Optic tract.* Transmission of visual impulses from the retina.[15] (p. 424), [19] (p. 399)

4. *Putamen.* Involved in motor function.[6] (p. 304), [7] (p. 11)

5. *Frontal lobe.* Involved in personality, insight, and foresight; initiation of voluntary movements; written and spoken language.[6] (pp. 18–20)

6. *Corpus callosum.* Interconnects the cerebral hemispheres.[2] (p. 131), [12] (p. 248), [16] (p. 33), [21] (p. 4)

7. *Interhemispheric (longitudinal) fissure.* Separates the cerebral hemispheres.[12] (p. 218), [19] (p. 257)

8. *Superior frontal gyrus.* Participates in the control and initiation of voluntary movements and is involved in personality, insight, and judgment.[6] (pp. 18–20), [18] (p. 674), [19] (p. 260)

9. *Precentral gyrus.* Location of the primary motor cortex.[1] (pp. 157, 326–327)

10. *Anterior horn of the lateral ventricle.* Anterior ependymal-lined cavity.[1] (pp. 172–173), [11] (p. 283), [12] (pp. 253–256)

11. *Third ventricle.* Transmits cerebrospinal fluid from the lateral ventricles to the fourth ventricle.[5] (p. 103)

12. *Insular cortex.* Associated with visceral functions, and anteriorly contains the cortical gustatory (taste) area.[2] (p. 196), [12] (pp. 209–213), [19] (p. 294)

13. *Globus pallidus.* Involved in the control of movement.[6] (p. 306), [7] (p. 11), [20] (pp. 276–277)

14. *Ansa lenticularis.* Transmits neuronal connections.[2] (pp. 281–282)

15. *Fornix.* Efferent tract of the hippocampus projecting to the mamillary bodies.[11] (p. 276), [12] (pp. 268–269), [19] (p. 269)

16. *Odontoid process (dens) of axis (C2).* Serves as the pivot around which the atlas rotates.[4] (p. 273–274), [8] (pp. 129–130)

17. *Axis (C2).* Serves as the pivot for the atlas (C1).[4] (pp. 273–274), [8] (pp. 129–130)

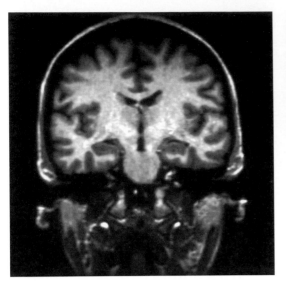

MRI

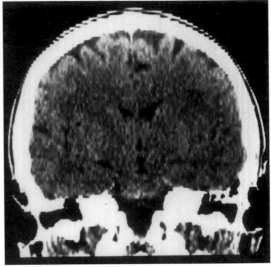

CT

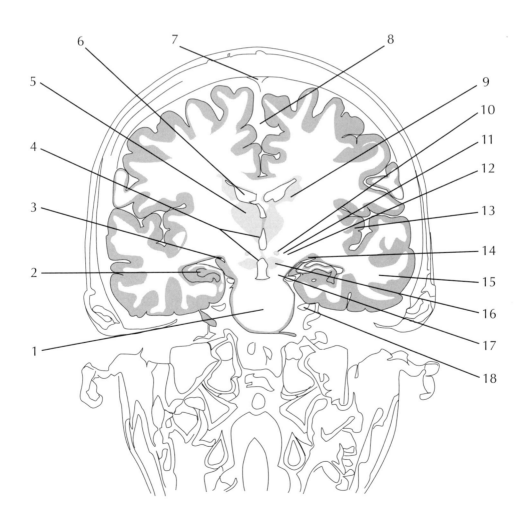

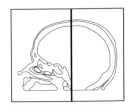

Coronal 11

1. *Pons.* Contains neural circuits that transmit information between the spinal cord and higher brain regions. Regulates levels of arousal, blood pressure, and respiration.[2 (p. 9), 11 (p. 181)]

2. *Dentate gyrus.* Involved in memory and the emotions related to survival.[2 (p. 379), 12 (pp. 266–267), 13 (pp. 325–326)]

3. *Choroid fissure.* Cerebrospinal fluid (CSF)-containing space, which forms a portion of the medial wall of the lateral ventricle.[1 (pp. 19, 172–173), 12 (pp. 255, 267)]

4. *Third ventricle.* Transmits CSF from the lateral ventricles to the fourth ventricle.[5 (p. 103)]

5. *Thalamus.* Serves as the main relay center for the nervous system.[6 (p. 234), 20 (pp. 258–262)]

6. *Anterior horn of the lateral ventricle.* Anterior ependymal-lined cavity.[1 (pp. 172–173), 11 (p. 283), 12 (pp. 253–256)]

7. *Superior sagittal sinus.* Drains blood from the brain and drains CSF from the subarachnoid space.[11 (pp. 292, 439)]

8. *Interhemispheric (longitudinal) fissure.* Separates the cerebral hemispheres.[12 (p. 218), 19 (p. 257)]

9. *Head of the caudate nucleus.* Involved in cognitive functions and movement.[6 (p. 304), 7 (p. 11), 12 (pp. 207–212), 15 (pp. 306–307), 18 (pp. 523–524)]

10. *Subthalamic nucleus.* Motor nucleus connected to the globus pallidus.[12 (pp. 193–194)]

11. *Subthalamus.* Involved in motor function and the regulation of drinking behaviors.[1 (pp. 149–150), 12 (pp. 193–194)]

12. *Cerebral peduncle.* Forms both sides of the midbrain, excluding the tectum.[2 (p. 226), 12 (p. 108)]

13. *Insular cortex.* Associated with visceral functions, and anteriorly contains the cortical gustatory (taste) area.[2 (p. 196), 12 (pp. 209–213), 19 (p. 294)]

14. *Tail of the caudate nucleus.* Involved in cognitive functions and movement.[6 (p. 304), 7 (p. 11), 12 (pp. 207–212), 15 (pp. 306–307), 18 (pp. 523–524)]

15. *Temporal lobe.* Involved in emotions, visceral responses, learning, and memory.[6 (pp. 21–22)]

16. *Red nucleus.* Relays impulses from the cerebral and cerebellar cortex to the spinal cord.[16 (pp. 435–436)]

17. *Basis pedunculi (crus cerebri).* Contains descending cortical fibers to the pyramids.[2 (pp. 224–225), 12 (p. 116)]

18. *Trigeminal nerve (cranial nerve V).* Provides sensation to the face, most of the scalp, the teeth, and the nasal and oral cavities. Also provides motor innervation of muscles of mastication.[1 (p. 404), 4 (p. 1059)]

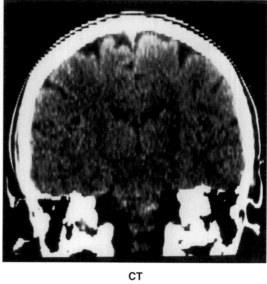

MRI

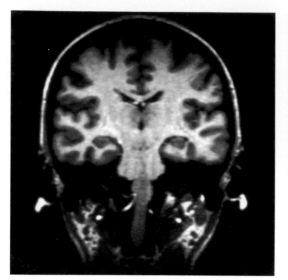

CT

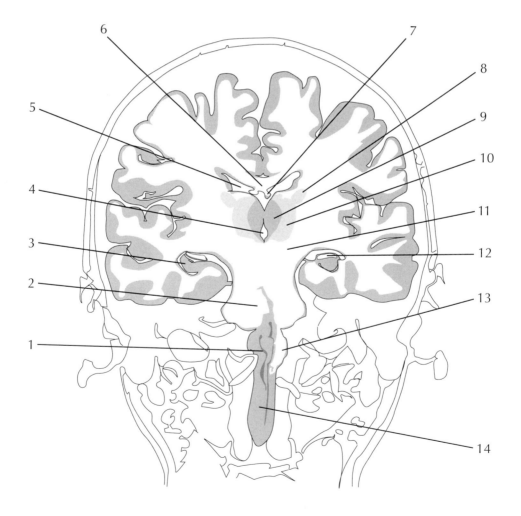

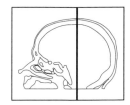

Coronal 12

1. *Medulla oblongata (myelencephalon or medulla).* Involved in digestion, breathing, blood pressure, and heart rate.[1] (pp. 15, 132–133), [2] (p. 9), [13] (pp. 7, 61), [15] (p. 9)

2. *Pons.* Contains neural circuits that transmit information between the spinal cord and higher brain regions. Regulates levels of arousal, blood pressure, and respiration.[2] (p. 9), [11] (p. 181)

3. *Dentate gyrus.* Involved in memory and the emotions related to survival.[2] (p. 379), [12] (pp. 266–267), [13] (pp. 353–354)

4. *Third ventricle.* Transmits cerebrospinal fluid (CSF) from the lateral ventricles to the fourth ventricle.[5] (p. 103)

5. *Anterior horn of the lateral ventricle.* Anterior ependymal-lined cavity.[1] (pp. 172–173), [11] (p. 283), [12] (pp. 253–256)

6. *Body of the corpus callosum.* Interconnects the cerebral hemispheres.[2] (pp. 51, 131), [12] (p. 248), [16] (p. 33)

7. *Fornix.* Efferent tract of the hippocampus projecting to the mamillary bodies.[11] (p. 276), [2] (pp. 268–269), [19] (p. 269)

8. *Lateral posterior nucleus.* Involved in relaying information from extrathalamic sources to the cerebral cortex.[1] (pp. 436–438), [22] (pp. 91–92)

9. *Dorsomedial nucleus.* Involved with memory and emotion.[12] (p. 184), [20] (p. 263)

10. *Centromedian nucleus.* Involved in consciousness and alertness, including the emotional response to painful stimuli.[12] (p. 184), [20] (p. 263)

11. *Cerebral peduncle.* Forms both sides of the midbrain, excluding the tectum.[2] (p. 226), [12] (p. 108)

12. *Choroid plexus.* Produces CSF.[5] (p. 102), [14] (p. 1213)

13. *Inferior olivary nucleus.* Involved in adaptive motor behavior.[1] (pp. 363–366), [6] (pp. 349–350)

14. *Pyramidal decussation.* Allows for one side of the brain to control the opposite side of the body.[12] (p. 336)

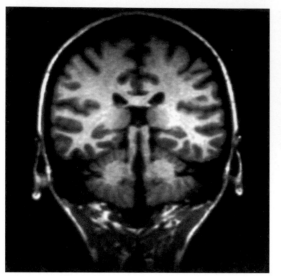

MRI

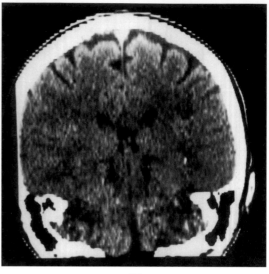

CT

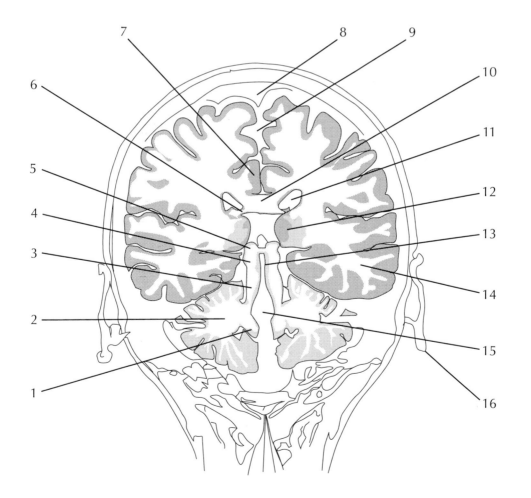

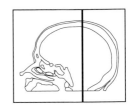

Coronal 13

1. *Inferior cerebellar peduncle.* Connects the cerebellum to the medulla, and is important in maintaining equilibrium.[2] (pp. 242, 249), [11] (p. 13), [12] (pp. 104–105), [20] (pp. 326–327)

2. *Middle cerebellar peduncle.* Connects cerebellum to pons, relaying input from the contralateral cerebral cortex to the lateral lobe of the cerebellum.[2] (pp. 242, 249), [11] (p. 13), [12] (pp. 104–105)

3. *Superior cerebellar peduncle.* Connects the cerebellum to the midbrain.[2] (pp. 242, 249), [11] (p. 13), [12] (pp. 104–105), [20] (p. 326)

4. *Inferior colliculus.* Participates in auditory pathways and relays impulses to the medial geniculate body.[2] (p. 178), [12] (p. 90), [20] (p. 372)

5. *Superior colliculus.* Receives visual signals directly from the retina or indirectly from the visual cortex and is essential for rapid eye movements.[1] (pp. 245–246, 412)

6. *Fornix.* Efferent tract of the hippocampus projecting to the mamillary bodies.[11] (p. 276), [12] (pp. 268–269), [19] (p. 269)

7. *Cingulate gyrus.* Plays a role in emotional behavior, the autonomic nervous system, learning, and memory.[12] (p. 272), [18] (pp. 255, 674)

8. *Superior sagittal sinus.* Drains blood from the brain and drains cerebrospinal fluid (CSF) from the subarachnoid space.[11] (pp. 292, 439)

9. *Interhemispheric (longitudinal) fissure.* Separates the cerebral hemispheres.[12] (p. 218), [19] (p. 257)

10. *Body of the corpus callosum.* Interconnects the cerebral hemispheres.[2] (pp. 51, 131), [12] (p. 248), [16] (p. 33)

11. *Lateral ventricle.* Ependymal-lined C-shaped cavity of each hemisphere filled with CSF.[11] (p. 183), [12] (pp. 253–256)

12. *Thalamus.* Serves as the main relay center for the nervous system.[6] (p. 234), [20] (pp. 258–263)

13. *Cerebral aqueduct (aqueduct of Sylvius).* Connects the third and fourth ventricles.[2] (p. 22), [11] (p. 213)

14. *Temporal lobe.* Involved in emotions, visceral responses, learning, and memory.[6] (pp. 21–22)

15. *Fourth ventricle.* Cavity filled with CSF.[7] (p. 70), [13] (p. 97)

16. *Lobule of the ear.* Inferior margin of the external ear.[4] (p. 1191)

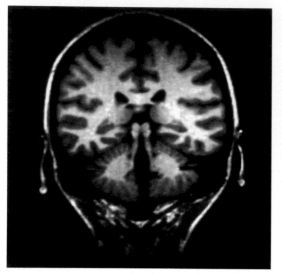

MRI

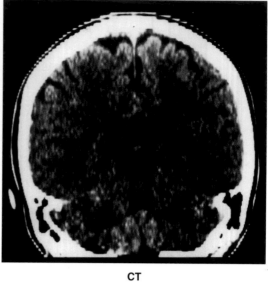

CT

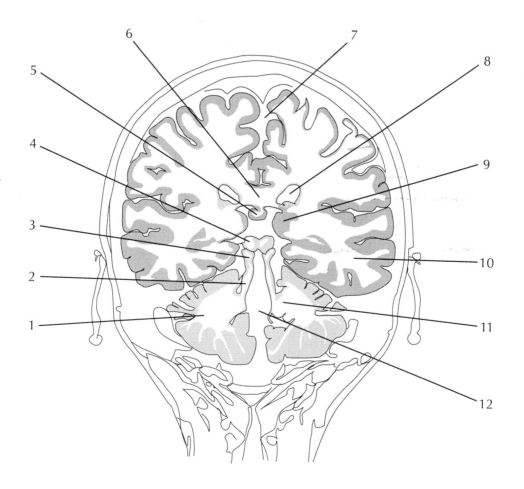

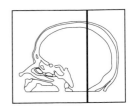

Coronal 14

1. *Cerebellum.* Primarily involved in motor function through the maintenance of equilibrium and the coordination of muscle action.[1] (pp. 15, 132–133), 4 (pp. 338–340), 6 (pp. 18–20)

2. *Superior cerebellar peduncle.* Connects the cerebellum to the midbrain.[2] (pp. 242, 249), 11 (p. 13), 12 (pp. 104–105), 20 (p. 326)

3. *Inferior colliculus.* Participates in auditory pathways and relays impulses to the medial geniculate body.[2] (p. 178), 12 (p. 90), 20 (p. 372)

4. *Superior colliculus.* Receives visual signals directly from the retina or indirectly from the visual cortex and is essential for rapid eye movements.[1] (pp. 245–246, 412)

5. *Pineal body.* Associated with the mechanisms that regulate circadian rhythm.[1] (p. 149), 8 (pp. 435–438)

6. *Body of the corpus callosum.* Interconnects the cerebral hemispheres.[2] (pp. 51, 131), 12 (p. 248), 16 (p. 33)

7. *Interhemispheric (longitudinal) fissure.* Separates the cerebral hemispheres.[12] (p. 218), 19 (p. 257)

8. *Lateral ventricle.* Ependymal-lined C-shaped cavity of each hemisphere filled with cerebrospinal fluid (CSF).[11] (p. 183), 12 (pp. 253–256)

9. *Pulvinar nucleus.* Along with the posterolateral and dorsolateral nuclei, forms the multimodal functional division of the thalamic nuclei.[3] (pp. 144–145), 22 (pp. 90–92)

10. *Temporal lobe.* Involved in emotions, visceral responses, learning, and memory.[6] (pp. 21–22)

11. *Middle cerebellar peduncle.* Connects cerebellum to pons, relaying input from the contralateral cerebral cortex to the lateral lobe of the cerebellum.[2] (pp. 242, 249), 11 (p. 13), 12 (pp. 104–105)

12. *Fourth ventricle.* Cavity filled with CSF.[7] (p. 70), 13 (p. 97)

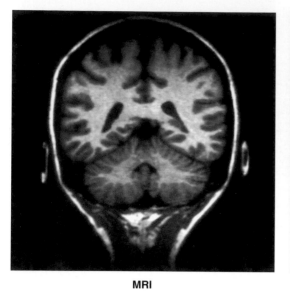

MRI

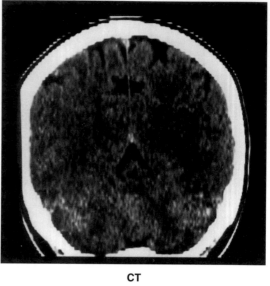

CT

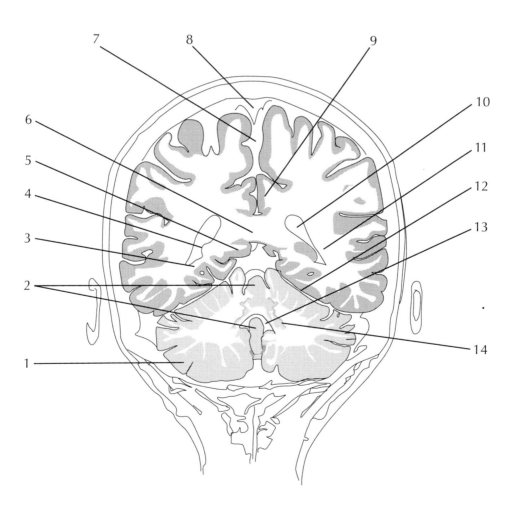

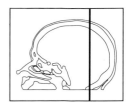

Coronal 15

1. *Cerebellum hemisphere.* Involved with movements of the extremities and fine coordinated movements.[3] (p. 283), [12] (p. 175), [15] (pp. 633–634)

2. *Cerebellar vermis.* Regulates and coordinates axial and girdle musculature. [3] (p. 282), [7] (p. 290)

3. *Fornix.* Efferent tract of the hippocampus projecting to the mamillary bodies.[11] (p. 276), [12] (pp. 268–269), [19] (p. 269)

4. *Calcar avis.* Formation caused by the calcarine fissure.[10] (pp. 74–75)

5. *Cingulate gyrus.* Plays a role in emotional behavior, the autonomic nervous system, learning, and memory.[12] (p. 272), [18] (pp. 255, 674)

6. *Splenium of the corpus callosum.* Enlargement of the corpus callosum posteriorly connecting the occipital lobes.[11] (pp. 244–245), [12] (p. 248), [19] (p. 269)

7. *Interhemispheric (longitudinal) fissure.* Separates the cerebral hemispheres.[12] (p. 218), [19] (p. 257)

8. *Superior sagittal sinus.* Drains blood from the brain and drains cerebrospinal fluid (CSF) from the subarachnoid space.[11] (pp. 292, 439)

9. *Cingulate gyrus.* Plays a role in emotional behavior, the autonomic nervous system, learning, and memory.[12] (p. 272), [18] (pp. 255, 674)

10. *Trigone of the lateral ventricle.* Where the body and temporal and occipital horns join to form a common cavity.[10] (pp. 74–75), [11] (p. 283), [12] (pp. 253–256)

11. *Optic radiation.* Maintains a precise visuotopic organization from the lateral geniculate body to the primary visual cortex.[1] (p. 240)

12. *Tentorium cerebelli.* Contains the dural sinuses, which provide venous drainage for the brain.[14] (p. 219)

13. *Fourth ventricle.* Cavity filled with CSF.[7] (p. 70), [13] (p. 97)

14. *Dentate nucleus.* Plays a role in somatic motor activity.[1] (pp. 353–354)

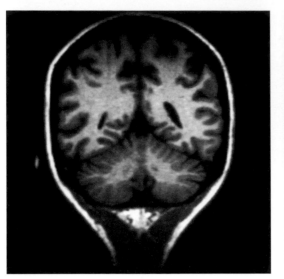

MRI

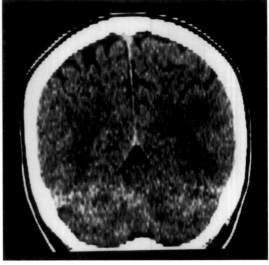

CT

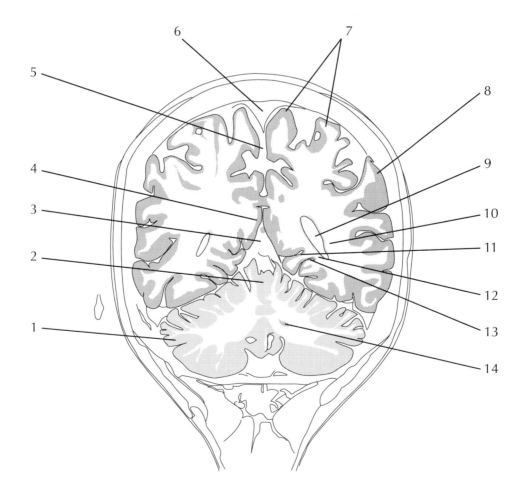

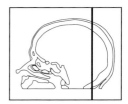

Coronal 16

1. *Cerebellar hemisphere.* Involved with movements of the extremities and fine coordinated movements.[3] (p. 283), [12] (p. 175), [15] (pp. 633–634)

2. *Cerebellar vermis.* Regulates and coordinates axial and girdle musculature.[3] (p. 282), [7] (p. 290)

3. *Straight venous sinus.* Provides cerebral venous drainage.[7] (p. 61), [22] (pp. 440–441)

4. *Cingulate gyrus.* Plays a role in emotional behavior, the autonomic nervous system, learning, and memory.[12] (p. 272), [18] (pp. 255, 674)

5. *Interhemispheric (longitudinal) fissure.* Separates the cerebral hemispheres.[12] (p. 218), [19] (p. 257)

6. *Superior sagittal sinus.* Drains blood from the brain and drains cerebrospinal fluid from the subarachnoid space.[11] (pp. 292, 439)

7. *Superior parietal lobule.* Involved in sensory appreciation such as stereognosis, graphesthesia, and two-point discrimination.[3] (p. 404), [12] (pp. 17–18), [14] (p. 886)

8. *Supramarginal gyrus.* Receives constructs of form, size, and body image from the somatosensory cortex; on the dominant side is involved in the comprehension of language.[3] (p. 404), [6] (pp. 18–20), [7] (pp. 405–407)

9. *Trigone of the lateral ventricle.* Where the body and temporal and occipital horns join to form a common cavity.[10] (pp. 74–75), [11] (p. 283), [12] (pp. 253–256)

10. *Optic radiation.* Maintains a precise visuotopic organization from the lateral geniculate body to the primary visual cortex.[1] (p. 240)

11. *Calcarine sulcus.* Marks the visual cortex.[11] (pp. 242, 260), [12] (pp. 217–218)

12. *Collateral eminence.* Shallow prominence secondary to the collateral fissure.[10] (pp. 74–75)

13. *Collateral sulcus.* Forms part of the lateral margin of the limbic association cortex.[2] (pp. 378–379)

14. *Dentate nucleus.* Plays a role in somatic motor activity.[1] (pp. 353–354)

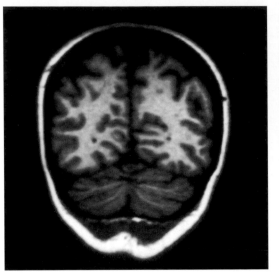

MRI

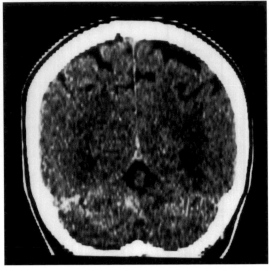

CT

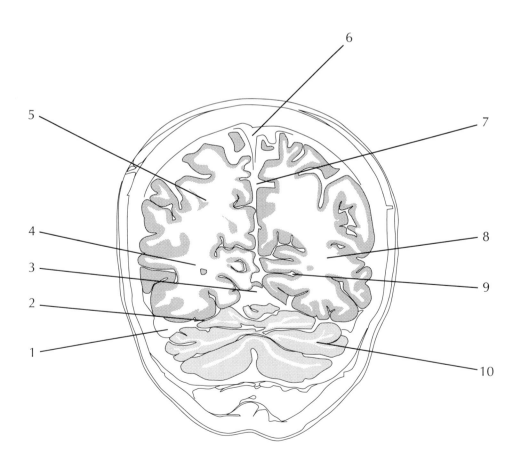

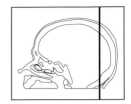

Coronal 17

1. *Transverse venous sinus.* Provides venous drainage for the brain.[1 (pp. 187–188), 25 (p. 251)]

2. *Tentorium cerebelli.* Contains the dural sinuses that provide venous drainage for the brain.[14 (p. 219)]

3. *Straight venous sinus.* Provides cerebral venous drainage.[7 (p. 61), 22 (pp. 440–441)]

4. *Optic radiation.* Maintains a precise visuo-topic organization from the lateral geniculate body to the primary visual cortex.[1 (p. 240)]

5. *Parietal lobe.* The postcentral gyrus is the first somesthetic area; however, it also has a motor component. The association cortex allows for processing the significance of sensory data, including prior experience.[9 (p. 693), 12 (pp. 232–235)]

6. *Superior sagittal sinus.* Drains blood from the brain and drains cerebrospinal fluid from the subarachnoid space.[11 (pp. 292, 439)]

7. *Interhemispheric (longitudinal) fissure.* Separates the cerebral hemispheres.[12 (p. 218), 19 (p. 257)]

8. *Occipital lobe.* Involved in the higher order processing of visual information.[6 (pp. 21–22)]

9. *Calcarine sulcus.* Marks the visual cortex.[11 (pp. 242, 260), 12 (pp. 217–218)]

10. *Cerebellum.* Primarily involved in motor function through the maintenance of equilibrium and the coordination of muscle action.[1 (pp. 15, 132–133), 4 (pp. 338–340), 6 (pp. 18–20)]

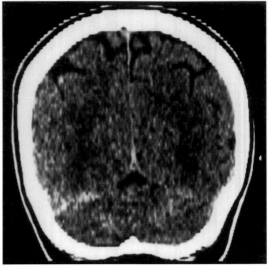

MRI

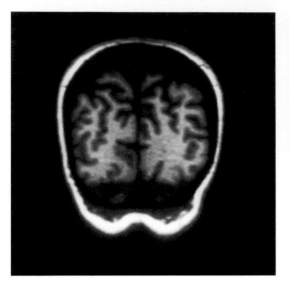

CT

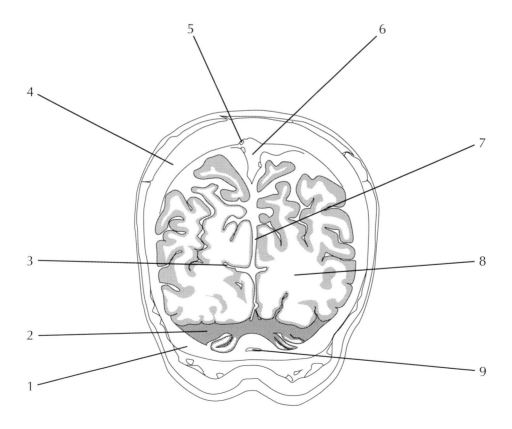

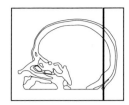

Coronal 18

1. *Squamous portion of occipital bone.* Provides protection for the underlying brain.[9] (p. 650)

2. *Transverse venous sinus.* Provides venous drainage for the brain.[1] (pp. 187–188), [25] (p. 251)

3. *Calcarine sulcus.* Marks the visual cortex.[11] (pp. 242, 260), [12] (pp. 217–218)

4. *Parietal bone.* Serves to enclose and protect the brain.[9] (p. 641), [24] (p. 170)

5. *Arachnoid granulations.* Clusters of arachnoid villi.[2] (p. 100)

6. *Superior sagittal sinus.* Drains blood from the brain and drains cerebrospinal fluid from the subarachnoid space.[11] (pp. 292, 439)

7. *Interhemispheric (longitudinal) fissure.* Separates the cerebral hemispheres.[12] (p. 218), [19] (p. 257)

8. *Occipital lobe.* Involved in the higher order processing of visual information.[6] (pp. 21–22)

9. *External occipital protuberance.* Forms the superior limit of the posterior aspect of the neck.[9] (p. 637)

3-D Images

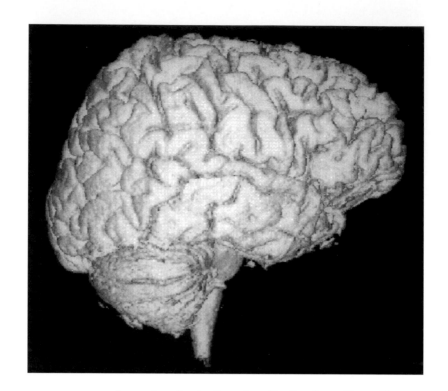

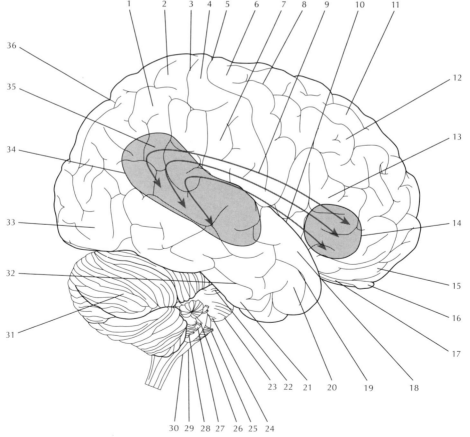

Brain: Lateral View

1. *Inferior parietal lobule.* May involve written, visual, and auditory language integration.[3] (p. 409), 6 (p. 20), 14 (p. 848)

2. *Superior parietal lobule.* Involved in sensory appreciation such as stereognosis, graphesthesia, and two-point discrimination.[3] (p. 404), 12 (pp. 17–28), 14 (p. 886)

3. *Postcentral sulcus.* Lies behind the postcentral gyrus.[6] (pp. 18–20)

4. *Postcentral gyrus.* The area of the cortex associated with general sensory information.[6] (pp. 18–20)

5. *Central sulcus.* Separates the primary motor cortex (frontal) from the primary somatosensory cortex (parietal).[19] (p. 257)

6. *Precentral gyrus.* Location of the primary motor cortex.[1] (pp. 157, 326–327)

7. *Supramarginal gyrus.* Receives constructs of form, size, and body image from the somatosensory cortex; on the dominant side is involved in the comprehension of language.[3] (p. 409), 6 (pp. 18–20), 7 (pp. 405–407)

8. *Precentral sulcus.* Anterior to the precentral gyrus.[6] (pp. 18–20)

9. *Arcuate fasciculus.* Connects Wernicke's and Broca's areas.[2] (p. 184)

10. *Sylvian fissure (lateral sulcus or fissure).* Separates temporal lobe from frontal and parietal lobes.[9] (pp. 257–258)

11. *Superior frontal gyrus.* Participates in the control and initiation of voluntary movements and is involved in personality, insight, and judgment.[6] (pp. 18–20), 18 (p. 674), 19 (p. 260)

12. *Middle frontal gyrus.* Participates in the control and initiation of voluntary movements; involved in personality, insight, and foresight.[6] (p. 18)

13. *Inferior frontal gyrus.* Important for the production of written and spoken language.[6] (p. 18)

14. *Broca's area.* Motor (expressive) speech area.[2] (p. 184)

15. *Orbital gyrus.* Involved in the conscious perception of odors.[1] (pp. 160, 296, 493)

16. *Olfactory bulb.* Receives projections of the olfactory nerves.[1] (p. 293)

17. *Olfactory tract.* Projects to the olfactory cortex.[1] (p. 294), 9 (p. 853)

18. *Superior temporal gyrus.* The primary auditory cortex.[1] (p. 161)

19. *Superior temporal sulcus.* Serves to separate the superior and middle temporal gyri.[1] (p. 161)

20. *Middle temporal gyrus.* Functions as one of the multimodal association areas.[22] (107)

21. *Inferior temporal gyrus.* Involved in the analysis of the form and color of visual stimuli.[2] (pp. 154–157), 12 (p. 219)

22. *Trigeminal nerve (cranial nerve V).* Provides sensation to the face, most of the scalp, the teeth, and the nasal and oral cavities. Also provides motor innervation to muscles of mastication.[1] (p. 404), 4 (p. 1059)

23. *Pons.* Contains neural circuits that transmit

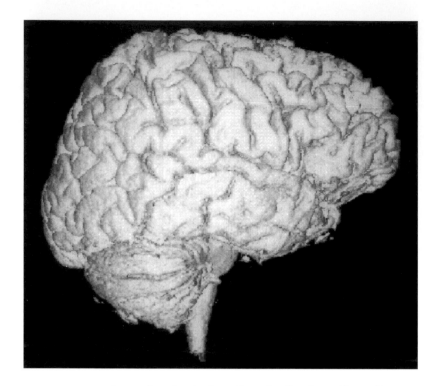

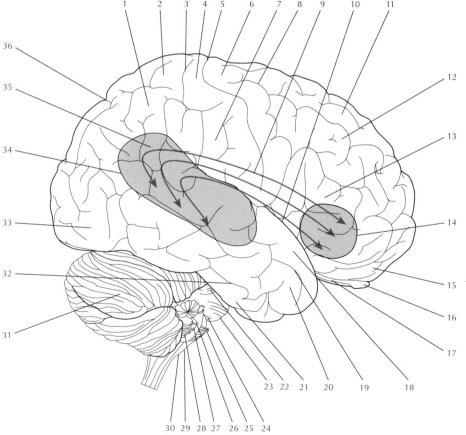

information between the spinal cord and higher brain regions. Regulates levels of arousal, blood pressure, and respiration.[2] (p. 9), [11] (p. 181)

24. *Abducens nerve (cranial nerve VI).* Lateral rectus muscle innervation (abduction).[1] (p. 104)

25. *Hypoglossal nerve (cranial nerve XII).* The motor nerve of the tongue providing innervation of the musculature.[1] (p. 429), [4] (p. 1083)

26. *Glossopharyngeal nerve (cranial nerve IX).* Innervates portions of the tongue and pharynx.[1] (p. 420), [20] (pp. 244–246)

27. *Vagus nerve.* Provides innervation to the thorax and abdomen, the pharynx and larynx, external ear, and taste buds on the epiglottis.[1] (p. 423), [4] (pp. 1076–1080)

28. *Accessory nerve (Spinal accessory nerve, cranial nerve XI).* Fibers from the motor neurons of the accessory nucleus and the nucleus ambiguus.[2] (pp. 322–330)

29. *Medulla oblongata (myelencephalon or medulla).* Involved in digestion, breathing, blood pressure, and heart rate.[1] (pp. 15, 132–133), [2] (p. 9), [13] (pp. 7, 61), [15] (p. 9)

30. *Olive.* Oval swelling of the ventral medulla produced by the inferior olivary complex. Involved in the coordination of learned movement.[2] (pp. 85–86, 96–99)

31. *Cerebellum.* Primarily involved in motor function through the maintenance of equilibrium and the coordination of muscle action.[1] (pp. 15, 132–133), [4] (pp. 399–340), [6] (pp. 18–20)

32. *Middle temporal sulcus.* Divides the middle and inferior temporal gyri.[1] (p. 161)

33. *Occipital lobe.* Involved in the higher order processing of visual information.[6] (pp. 21–22)

34. *Wernicke's area.* Important for the understanding of spoken or written language as well as gestures and musical sounds.[1] (p. 169)

35. *Angular gyrus.* On the dominant side is involved with the comprehension of language.[6] (pp. 18–20), [7] (pp. 405–407)

36. *Parietal occipital sulcus.* Separates the parietal and occipital lobes.[11] (p. 233), [19] (p. 259)

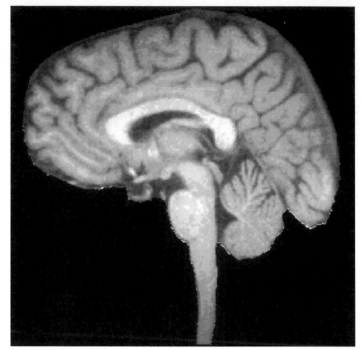

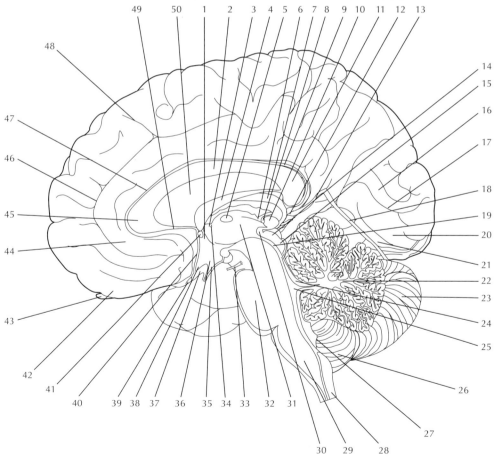

Brain: Medial View–Right

1. *Column of fornix.* Part of the myelinated pathway connecting the hippocampus with subcortical structures.[11 (p. 276), 12 (pp. 268–269), 19 (p. 269)]

2. *Body of corpus callosum.* Interconnects the cerebral hemispheres.[2 (pp. 51, 131), 12 (p. 248), 16 (p. 33)]

3. *Foramen of Monro.* Connections between the paired lateral ventricle and the unpaired midline third ventricle.[1 (p. 172)]

4. *Fornix.* Efferent tract of the hippocampus projecting to the mamillary bodies.[11 (p. 276), 12 (pp. 268–269), 19 (p. 269)]

5. *Massa intermedia (interthalamic adhesion).* A midline nucleus of the thalamus, which joins the two thalami medially, but without direct fiber connections across the midline.[1 (pp. 151, 433)]

6. *Habenular nuclei.* Influences the hypothalamus.[3 (p. 165), 12 (pp. 194–195)]

7. *Crus of the fornix.* Part of the myelinated pathway that connects the hippocampus with subcortical structures.[11 (p. 276), 12 (pp. 268–269), 19 (p. 269)]

8. *Habenular commissure.* Contains fibers of the stria medullaris thalami with interconnections between the habenular nuclei.[3 (p. 165), 12 (pp. 194–195)]

9. *Indusium griseum.* Covers the dorsal surface of the body of the corpus callosum.[12 (p. 248)]

10. *Pineal gland.* Associated with the mechanisms that regulate circadian rhythm.[1 (p. 149), 8 (pp. 435–438)]

11. *Splenium of the corpus callosum.* Enlargement of the corpus callosum posteriorly connecting the occipital lobes.[11 (pp. 244–245), 12 (p. 248), 19 (269)]

12. *Internal cerebral veins.* Formed from the thalamostriate and the choroid veins and forming the great cerebral vein (vein of Galen).[11 (p. 455)]

13. *Great cerebral vein (vein of Galen).* Assists in venous drainage of the brain.[10 (pp. 275–294)]

14. *Superior colliculus.* Receives visual signals directly from the retina or indirectly from the visual cortex, and is essential for rapid eye movements.[1 (pp. 245–246, 412)]

15. *Inferior colliculus.* Participates in auditory pathways and relays impulses to the medial geniculate body.[2 (p. 178), 20 (p. 372)]

16. *Cuneus.* Constitutes part of the primary visual cortex.[1 (pp. 160–161)]

17. *Calcarine sulcus.* Marks the visual cortex.[11 (pp. 242, 260), 12 (pp. 217–218)]

18. *Straight venous sinus.* Provides cerebral venous drainage.[7 (p. 61), 22 (pp. 440–441)]

19. *Cerebral aqueduct.* Connects the third and fourth ventricles.[2 (p. 22), 11 (p. 213)]

20. *Cingulate gyrus.* Plays a role in emotional behavior, the autonomic nervous system, learning, and memory.[12 (p. 272), 18 (pp. 255, 674)]

21. *Fusiform gyrus.* Involved in the storage and recall of visual memories.[12 (pp. 235–236), 14 (p. 674)]

22. *Cerebellar vermis.* Regulates and coordinates axial and girdle musculature.[3 (p. 282), 7 (p. 290)]

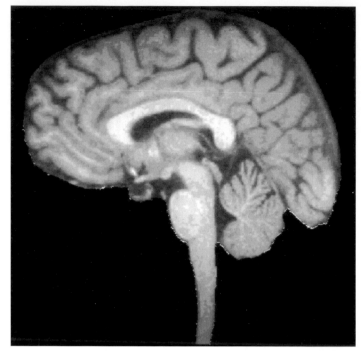

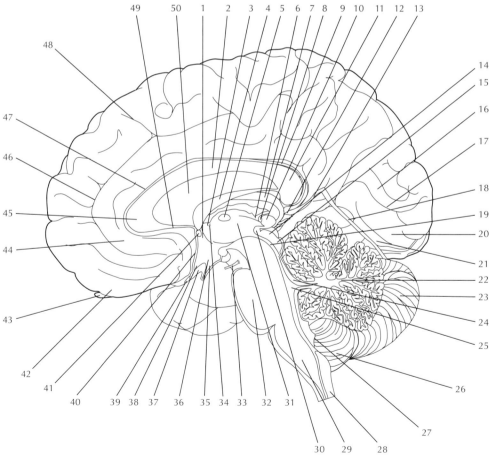

23. *Cerebellar hemisphere.* Involved with movement of the extremities and fine coordinated movements.[3 (p. 283), 12 (p.175), 15 (pp. 633–634)]

24. *Superior medullary velum.* Forms part of the roof of the fourth ventricle.[1 (pp. 136–137)]

25. *Fourth ventricle.* Cavity filled with cerebrospinal fluid (CSF).[7 (p. 70), 13 (p. 97)]

26. *Cerebellar tonsil.* Concerned with guiding limb movement and posture.[2 (p. 242)]

27. *Foramen of Magendie.* Outlet of the ventricular system to the subarachnoid space.[1 (p. 174), 14 (p. 117)]

28. *Spinal cord.* Innervates the motor and sensory areas of the body.[1 (p. 117), 4 (p. 864)]

29. *Medulla oblongata (myelencephalon or medulla).* Involved in digestion, breathing, blood pressure, and heart rate.[1 (pp. 15, 132–133), 2 (p. 9), 13 (pp. 7, 61), 15 (p. 9)]

30. *Posterior commissure.* Contains collections of nerve cells that include pupillary light reflex involvement.[11 (p. 246), 12 (p. 195)]

31. *Thalamus.* Serves as the main relay center for the nervous system.[6 (p. 234), 20 (pp. 258–263)]

32. *Pons.* Contains neural circuits that transmit information between the spinal cord and higher brain regions. Regulates levels of arousal, blood pressure, and respiration.[2 (p. 9), 11 (p. 181)]

33. *Oculomotor nerve (cranial nerve III).* Innervates four of the six extraocular muscles as well as the levator palpebrae.[2 (pp. 322–333), 25 (p. 189)]

34. *Choroid plexus of third ventricle.* Produces CSF.[5 (p. 102), 14 (p. 1213)]

35. *Infundibular recess.* CSF-filled recess in the floor of the third ventricle.[2 (p. 350)]

36. *Hypothalamus.* Regulates the autonomic nervous system and also controls pituitary function.[3 (pp. 421–424)]

37. *Optic chiasm.* Convergence of the optic nerves.[2 (p. 143), 11 (p. 227)]

38. *Optic recess.* Anterior projection of the third ventricle.[3 (p. 315)]

39. *Optic nerve.* Nerve of sight.[7 (pp. 221, 227)]

40. *Lamina terminalis.* Provides input to the hypothalamus regarding blood volume and blood pressure control.[2 (pp. 36, 356), 12 (pp. 196–197)]

41. *Anterior commissure.* A neocortical "corpus callosum."[11 (p. 246), 12 (pp. 249–250)]

42. *Lateral orbital gyrus.* May be involved in such processes as personality, insight, and foresight.[1 (p. 444), 2 (pp. 154–160)]

43. *Olfactory bulb.* Receives projections of the olfactory nerves.[1 (p. 293)]

44. *Cingulate gyrus.* Plays a role in emotional behavior, the autonomic nervous system, learning, and memory.[12 (p. 272), 18 (pp. 255, 674)]

45. *Genu of corpus callosum.* Connects the frontal lobes.[2 (pp. 51, 131), 12 (p. 248), 15 (p. 365), 19 (p. 269)]

46. *Cingulate sulcus.* Separates the cingulate gyrus from the superior frontal gyrus.[19 (p. 261)]

47. *Callosal sulcus.* Separates the cingulate gyrus from the corpus callosum.[11 (p. 236)]

48. *Paracentral sulcus.* A branch of the cingulate sulcus.[12 (pp. 221–222)]

49. *Rostrum of the corpus callosum.* Forms the anterior wall of the third ventricle.[2 (p. 229), 12 (p. 148)]

50. *Septum pellucidum.* Forms the medial wall of the body and anterior horns of the lateral ventricle.[2 (p. 384), 12 (pp. 249–250), 19 (p. 273)]

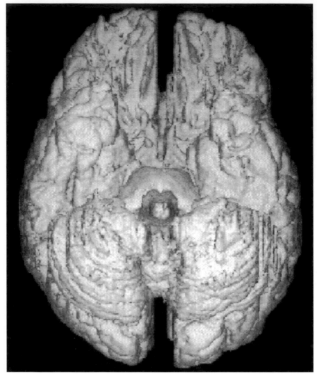

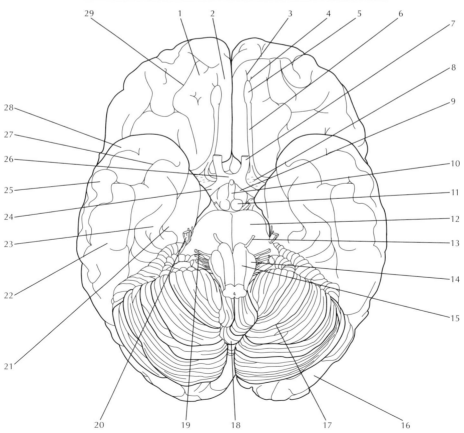

Brain: Basal View

1. *Orbital gyrus.* Involved in the conscious perception of odors.[1] (pp. 160, 296, 493)

2. *Lateral orbital gyrus of the frontal lobe (gyrus rectus, straight gyrus).* May be involved in such processes as personality, insight, and foresight.[6] (pp. 18–20), [22] (p. 104)

3. *Olfactory sulcus.* Forms the lateral margin of the gyrus rectus.[1] (p. 160)

4. *Olfactory nerve (cranial nerve I).* The nerve of smell.[9] (p. 853)

5. *Olfactory bulb.* Receives projections of the olfactory nerves.[1] (p. 293)

6. *Olfactory tract.* Projects to the olfactory cortex.[1] (p. 294), [9] (p. 853)

7. *Optic nerve (cranial nerve II).* Nerve of sight.[7] (pp. 221, 227)

8. *Anterior perforated substance.* Contains the olfactory tubercle.[2] (pp. 200–202)

9. *Tuber cinereum.* A swelling that has most of the hypothalamic nuclei that regulate the release of the anterior pituitary hormones.[2] (p. 350), [12] (p. 196)

10. *Infundibulum (pituitary stalk, hypophyseal stalk).* Connects the pituitary gland to the hypothalamus.[2] (p. 355), [12] (p. 196), [15] (p. 739)

11. *Mamillary body.* Receives hippocampal input.[1] (p. 386), [2] (pp. 367–368, 381, 392)

12. *Pons.* Contains neural circuits that transmit information between the spinal cord and higher brain regions. Regulates levels of arousal, blood pressure, and respiration.[2] (p. 9), [11] (p. 181)

13. *Trochlear nerve (cranial nerve IV).* In-nervates the superior oblique muscle for movement of the eye down and out.[1] (p. 410)

14. *Olive.* Oval swelling of the ventral medulla produced by the inferior olivary complex. Involved in the coordination of learned movement.[12] (pp. 85–86, 96–99)

15. *Pyramid.* Contains the lateral and ventral corticospinal tracts and the corticobulbar tracts.[2] (p. 229)

16. *Occipital pole.* Part of the primary visual cortex.[11] (p. 265)

17. *Cerebellar hemisphere.* Involved with movements of the extremities and fine coordinated movements.[3] (p. 283), [12] (p. 176), [15] (pp. 633–634)

18. *Cerebellar vermis.* Regulates and coordinates axial and girdle musculature.[3] (p. 282), [7] (p. 290)

19. *Accessory nerve (spinal accessory nerve, cranial nerve XI).* Fibers from the motor neurons of the accessory nucleus and the nucleus ambiguus.[2] (pp. 322–330)

20. *Trigeminal nerve (cranial nerve V).* Provides sensation to the face, most of the scalp, the teeth, and the nasal and oral cavities. Also provides motor innervation to muscles of mastication.[1] (p. 404), [4] (p. 1059)

21. *Parahippocampal gyrus.* Involved in olfactory and memory perceptions.[2] (pp. 200–202), [15] (pp. 306–307)

22. *Inferior temporal gyrus.* Involved in the analysis of the form and color of visual stimuli.[2] (pp. 154–157), [12] (p. 219)

23. *Fusiform gyrus (lateral occipitotemporal*

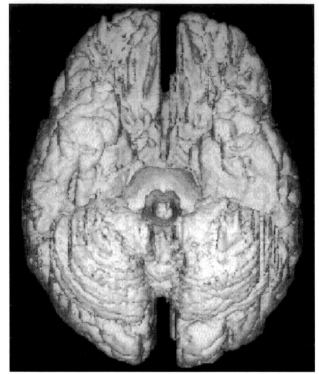

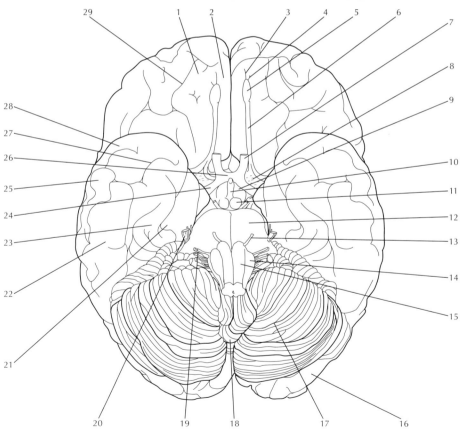

gyrus). Involved in the storage and recall of visual memories.[12 (pp. 235–236), 14 (p. 674)]

24. *Optic tract.* Transmission of visual impulses from the retina.[15 (p. 424), 19 (p. 399)]

25. *Middle temporal gyrus.* Functions as one of the multimodal association areas.[22 (p. 107)]

26. *Optic chiasm.* Convergence of the optic nerves.[2 (p. 143), 11 (p. 227)]

27. *Middle temporal sulcus.* Divides the middle and inferior temporal gyri.[1 (p. 161)]

28. *Superior temporal gyrus.* The primary auditory gyrus.[1 (p. 161)]

29. *Orbital sulcus.* Forms the lateral margin of the margin of the lateral gyrus.[1 (pp. 159–161)]

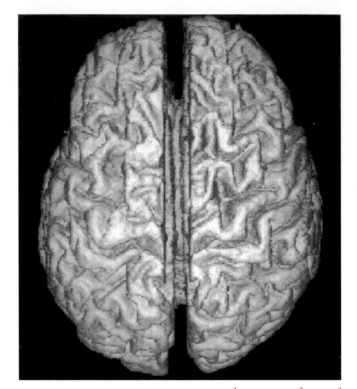

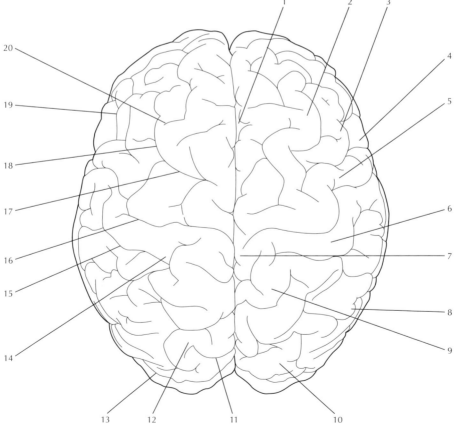

Brain: Axial View

1. *Interhemispheric (longitudinal) fissure.* Separates the cerebral hemisphere.[12] (p. 218), [19] (p. 257)

2. *Superior frontal gyrus.* Participates in the control and initiation of voluntary movements and is involved in personality, insight, and judgment.[6] (pp. 18–20), [18] (p. 674), [19] (p. 260)

3. *Middle frontal gyrus.* Participates in the control and initiation of voluntary movements; involved in personality, insight, and foresight.[6] (p. 18)

4. *Inferior frontal gyrus.* Important for the production of written and spoken language.[6] (p. 18)

5. *Precentral gyrus.* Location of the primary motor cortex.[1] (pp. 157, 326–327)

6. *Postcentral gyrus.* The area of the cortex associated with general sensory information.[6] (pp. 18–20)

7. *Paracentral lobule.* Medial extension of the precentral (motor) and postcentral (sensory) gyri.[6] (pp. 18–20)

8. *Inferior parietal lobule.* May involve written, visual, and auditory language integration.[3] (p. 409), [6] (p. 20), [14] (p. 848)

9. *Superior parietal lobule.* Involved in sensory appreciation, such as stereognosis, graphesthesia, and two-point discrimination.[3] (p. 404), [12] (pp. 17–18), [14] (p. 886)

10. *Occipital pole.* Part of the primary visual cortex.[11] (p. 265)

11. *Parietal occipital sulcus.* Separates the parietal and occipital lobes.[11] (p. 233), [19] (p. 259)

12. *Occipital lobe.* Involved in the higher order processing of visual information.[6] (pp. 21–22)

13. *Occipital sulcus.* Forms the lateral margin of the lateral gyrus.[1] (pp. 159–161)

14. *Parietal lobe.* The postcentral gyrus is the first somesthetic area; however, it also has a motor component. The association cortex allows for processing the significance of sensory data, including prior experience.[9] (p. 693), [12] (pp. 232–235)

15. *Postcentral sulcus.* Lies behind the postcentral gyrus.[6] (pp. 18–20)

16. *Central sulcus.* Separates the primary motor cortex (frontal) from the primary somatosensory cortex (parietal).[19] (p. 257)

17. *Precentral sulcus.* Anterior to the precentral gyrus.[6] (pp. 18–20)

18. *Superior frontal sulcus.* Separates the superior frontal gyrus from the middle frontal gyrus.[12] (p. 219)

19. *Inferior frontal sulcus.* Divides the lateral surface of the frontal lobe.[12] (p. 219)

20. *Frontal lobe.* Involved in personality, insight, and foresight; initiation of voluntary movement; written and spoken language.[6] (pp. 18–20)

References

1. Gray H, Goss, CM. *Anatomy of the Human Body*, 28th ed. Lea & Febiger, Philadelphia, 1966.
2. Martin JH. *Neuroanatomy Text and Atlas*. Elsevier Science Publishing, New York, 1989.
3. Hayman LA, Hinck VA. *Clinical Brain Imaging, Normal Structure and Functional Anatomy*. Mosby-Year Book, St. Louis, 1992.
4. Williams P, Warwick R. *Gray's Anatomy*, 36th ed. W.B. Saunders, Philadelphia, 1980.
5. Hodges FJ III. Anatomy of the ventricles and subarachnoid spaces. *Semin Roentgenol* 5:101–121, 1970.
6. Nolte J. *The Human Brain: An Introduction to Its Functional Anatomy*, 2nd ed. C.V. Mosby, St. Louis, 1988.
7. Noback CR, Strominger NL, Demarest RJ. *The Human Nervous System, Introduction and Review,* 4th ed. Lea & Febiger, Philadelphia, 1991.
8. Crouch JE. *Functional Human Anatomy*, 4th ed. Lee & Febiger, Philadelphia, 1985.
9. Moore KL. *Clinically Oriented Anatomy*, 3rd ed. Williams & Wilkins, Baltimore, 1992.
10. Wilson M. *The Anatomic Foundation of Neuroradiology of the Brain*, 2nd ed. Little, Brown, Boston, 1972.
11. Snell RS. *Clinical Neuroanatomy for Medical Students*. Little, Brown, Boston, 1980.
12. Barr ML, Kieman JA. *The Human Nervous System: An Anatomical Viewpoint*, 5th ed. J.B. Lippincott, Philadelphia, 1983.
13. Heimer L. *The Human Brain and Spinal Cord, Functional Neuroanatomy and Dissection Guide*. Springer-Verlag, New York, 1983.
14. *Dorland's Illustrated Medical Dictionary*, 25th ed. W.B. Saunders, Philadelphia, 1974.
15. Kandel ER, Schwartz JH, Jessel TM. *Principles of Neural Science*, 3rd ed. Elsevier Science Publishing, New York, 1991.
16. Carpenter MB, Sutin J. *Human Neuroanatomy*, 8th ed. Williams & Wilkins, Baltimore, 1983.
17. Moore KL. *Clinically Oriented Anatomy*, 2nd ed. Williams & Wilkins, Baltimore, 1985.
18. Kandel ER, Schwartz JH. *Principles of Neural Science*, 2nd ed. Elsevier Science Publishing, New York, 1985.
19. Snell RS. *Clinical Neuroanatomy for Medical Students*, 2nd ed. Little, Brown, Boston, 1987.
20. House EL, Pansky B. *A Functional Approach to Neuroanatomy*, 2nd ed. McGraw-Hill, New York, 1967.
21. Liebman M. *Neuroanatomy Made Easy and Understandable*, 3rd ed. Aspen Publishers, Rockville, MD, 1986.
22. deGroot J, Chusid JG. *Correlative Neuroanatomy*, 20th ed. Appleton and Lange, Norwalk, CT, 1988.
23. Snell RS, *Clinical Anatomy for Medical Students*, 2nd ed. Little, Brown and Company, Boston, 1981.
24. Luciano DS, Vander AJ, Sherman JH. *Human Anatomy and Physiology: Structure and Function*. McGraw-Hill, New York, 1983.
25. Orrison WW Jr. *Introduction to Neuroimaging*. Little, Brown, Boston, 1989.
26. Nieuwenhuys R, Voogd J, Van Huijzen C. *The Human Central Nervous System (A Synopsis and Atlas)*. Springer-Verlag, Berlin, 1978.

Index

(The page numbers set in bold type denote when the term is defined, otherwise the term has been referenced in another term's definition.)